HOSPITAL HEALTH EDUCATION

A Guide to Program Development

Donald J. Breckon, M.P.H., Ph.D.
Central Michigan University

AN ASPEN PUBLICATION®
Aspen Systems Corporation
Rockville, Maryland
London
1982

Library of Congress Cataloging in Publication Data

Breckon, Donald J.
Hospital health education.

Bibliography: p. 267
Includes index.
1. Patient education. 2. Health education.
3. Hospital care. 4. Hospital and community. I. Title.
[DNLM: 1. Health education. 2. Patient education.
3. Hospital administration. WX 158.5 B829h]
RA775.5.P38B73 610′.7 82-1664
ISBN: 0-89443-681-3 AACR2

Library of Congress Catalog Card Number: 82-1664
ISBN: 0-89443-681-3

Printed in the United States of America

1 2 3 4 5

Table of Contents

Preface

This book presents issues of importance to the education and practice of hospital health educators. My primary objective is to provide direction and assistance to those responsible for planning, implementing, and evaluating a health education program in a hospital setting. The book focuses on the hospital's role in providing health education activities for patients and their families, the community in which the hospital is located, and hospital employees. Health education for the staff should not be confused with more commonplace "inservice" or "continuing education" activities. Rather, as presented in these pages, these specialized programs are geared to improve the health of hospital staff members.

This book is designed as a practical guide. Because hospital health education is a new and growing specialty, I offer a number of pragmatic suggestions, outlining "what to do" and "how to do it." Some recommendations practitioners will want to adopt as is; other examples and pieces of practical advice, I present as starting points to be adapted to fit the needs of particular programs or refined by individual health care professionals.

Donald J. Breckon
April 1982

Acknowledgments

I want to acknowledge formally the many ways that my students in Central Michigan University's Patient Education Programming classes have assisted me over the years. Each time I teach the course, it seems that I learn more than I teach. The diverse background of the students and the perspectives they bring to the class have been of enormous value. Since many are employed in a hospital setting, countless opportunities exist to experiment with innovative ideas and to report back on what has worked and why. The reading, thinking, and writing that students have performed for class assignments have contributed enormously to the breadth and depth of my knowledge. The most exciting facet of patient education classes has always been when class members and the professor engage in a discussion leading to the charting of new ground for both. Such has occurred in my classes on numerous occasions.

To the students in the many sections of that class I say—"Thank you. This book is dedicated to you."

Part I

An Overview

part I

Hospital health education is an emerging discipline. It has roots in antiquity, having been applied in varying forms by diverse practitioners of the medical arts. Today, with health care institutions required to provide programs, health education is becoming a highly specialized field. It has evolved from early practices of "answering questions" and "telling patients what they ought to do," to well-planned, implemented, and evaluated programs that use adult learning theory, behavioral change programs, and sophisticated technology in ways that have been documented to improve patient prognosis. It has changed from focusing on the health of the individual patient to concentrating on the health of the hospital staff and members of the community at large.

As with other new disciplines, hospital health education is changing and growing rapidly, causing some confusion and misunderstanding. Surprisingly, some hospital personnel have never heard of the field. Others have limited or inaccurate perceptions, while few staffers have been able to keep up with the state of the art.

Due to the originality of the field, it is especially important to provide some common understanding of the foundations of the discipline. Part I will review the basics, providing a foundation to discuss planning and delivery of a hospital health education program.

Chapter 1

Hospital Health Education: An Historical Perspective*

---

* Adapted from Donald J. Breckon, "Highlights in the Evolution of Hospital-Based Patient Education Programs," *Journal of Allied Health,* Summer 1976, by permission of Charles Slack Inc., © 1976.

1

INTRODUCTION

The classic concept of a hospital treating only the very sick is rapidly disappearing. Similarly, hospitals no longer care only for those near death. Instead, they are becoming centers for preventive medicine.

In the mid-1970s, about 97 percent of the United States' health care dollar was spent on treatment rather than on prevention.[1] However, this pattern is changing, and the rate of change seems to be escalating. Many hospitals have committed a significant amount of resources to prevention and others are ready to follow that lead. The concept of preventive medicine is becoming widely accepted, even if this emphasis is not yet reflected in institutional budgets.

Hospital-based preventive medicine is beginning to rely more heavily on the educational process. Professionals have long been aware that most of the chronic illnesses being treated involve lifestyle and personal choice factors. Health education has been addressing such personal risk factors with varying degrees of success. For example, patients with coronary heart disease or cerebralvascular disease have shown decreasing mortality rates, in part due to the decreased consumption of saturated fats,[2] the decreased incidence of cigarette smoking among men,[3] and the dramatic increase in jogging. Some of the credit for these advances can be attributed to health education programs.

Another major concern of health care professionals has been patient behavior after discharge. One compliance study revealed that between 15 and 95 percent of orders by physicians were ignored with resultant relapse and readmission.[4] Again, one of the major causative factors was a lack of understanding of what was to be done and why it was important. To help remedy this situation, experimental educational programs were implemented and were found to increase compliance and reduce readmission.[5] Such programs were popularly called patient education programs and were replicated in many progressive hospitals. In fact, a 1978 survey revealed that more than 2,921 hospitals had operational patient education programs.[6]

EARLY DEVELOPMENTS

Patient education is as old as the doctor-patient relationship. Most doctors have long recognized the importance of the patient's understanding of necessary activities to regain and retain health. While some physicians have emphasized this more than others, the doctor-patient relationship has always had an educational component, similar to the nurse-patient relationship. Frequently, the role of the nurse in teaching was even greater than that of the doctor, including, but not limited to, the answering of specific questions raised by patients.

As the knowledge explosion increased, patients also became more sophisticated and demanded to know more about their problems than ever before. This was magnified by consumerism, the women's health movement, and the larger self-care movement. It also received impetus from court decisions affirming a patient's legal right to know. "Informed consent" became a major issue for medical staff; more explanation and justification were required of medical staff than in previous years. This widespread "health consciousness" was bringing more people with a greater desire to know to doctors' offices. Yet, because of increased loads, physicians had less time to spend with each patient to explain treatment.

Another of the primary factors responsible for the increased emphasis on patient education was the development of prepaid health care groups, such as, the Health Insurance Plan of Greater New York, the Kaiser Permanente Plan, and the Group Health Cooperative Program. For a monthly fee, families were entitled to complete medical care, both in and out of the hospital. When health insurance groups were faced with the necessity of paying the total cost of medical care, it became apparent that prevention and informed self-care could reduce the total health care bill. These early groups were among the first to implement hospital-based patient education programs.

References in Publications

References to patient education first began to appear in the literature during the 1950s. Articles appeared in publications of the Veterans Administration (VA)[7] which, like the prepaid groups already mentioned, was delegated to provide total medical care. The VA was therefore more willing to reduce long-range patient care costs through educational efforts.

Other references to patient education appeared in a variety of publications.[8–12] These attempts at disseminating the concept to other professionals were largely responsible for the growth of interest in the field and recognition of patient education as an integral feature of health care.

The staffs of several prepaid health care programs met jointly for an annual meeting throughout the 1950s, but the Tenth Annual Group Health Institute, held in 1960 and whose proceedings were widely distributed, was especially significant in spreading the concept of patient education.[13] Ross Laboratories, publishers of a monthly newsletter directed toward hospital administrators, devoted its entire August 1963 issue to "Health Education in a Hospital Setting." The issue concluded by stating:

> The hospital has the opportunity to teach constructive health habits. The effectiveness of a hospital's health education efforts can be measured by the number of persons it succeeds in rehabilitating to useful lives, and the number of readmissions it succeeds in preventing.[14]

COORDINATING THE EFFORTS

In 1964 the American Hospital Association (AHA) sponsored a conference in Chicago entitled "Health Education in the Hospital" whose proceedings became an important reference. The participants agreed that hospitals should provide patient education to the fullest extent possible and urged the establishment of demonstration programs and staff inservice training programs. They further recommended that the AHA should act as the nationwide agency to stimulate development of patient education programs.[15] The acceptance of an advocacy role by this organization was an important milestone in the evolution of patient education programs. Significantly the conference was funded by the Metropolitan Life Insurance Company, a private insurance company endorsing the concept.

Representing another segment of society, the Russell Sage Foundation also became involved in helping patient education gain acceptance. This private philanthropic organization, long committed to health and social welfare programs, commissioned the writing and publication of a series of three monographs later published in book form.[16] This work is still frequently referenced, attesting to its importance and farsightedness.

In the 1966 leaflet entitled *Hospitals as Education Institutions* the AHA endorsed a policy of patient education. It, too, has been a significant step forward in the effort to legitimize patient education programs.

Yet another segment of the nation's health care system officially entered the struggle in 1968 when the American Public Health Association (Public Health Education Section) appointed a Committee on Educational Tasks in Chronic Illness. The committee concluded that patient education was an integral part of patient care. Members went on to urge the use of the "team approach" in patient education consisting of the physician, the nurse, and the education specialist. The committee further urged the use of a written "educational prescription" that would be part of patients' permanent health records.[17] The Committee developed the following five-step model:

1. Identify the educational needs of the patient and family,
2. Establish educational goals for the patient and family,
3. Select appropriate educational methods,
4. Carry out the educational programs, and
5. Evaluate the patient and family education.[18]

The elaboration of each step gave specific practical information. Published as a monograph, this was the first "cookbook approach" for those who wanted to perform patient education. It was expanded and updated in 1979 and continues to be made available.

The 1960s were also important in producing a review of the research-to-date on patient education.[19] In 1968 the Society of Public Health Education produced the most comprehensive review up to that time of current literature.

ESTABLISHMENT OF CREDIBILITY

In September 1971 President Richard Nixon appointed a committee to study health education nationwide. Consisting of 16 people representing a wide range of interests, inside and outside the health care field, the President's Committee on Health Education was charged with recommending a new rational approach to health education.

Holding hearings around the nation, the committee found little effective health education for patients in hospitals. Yet it also determined that a hospital stay was one of the junctures during health care when the patient and his/her family were most susceptible to education. The Committee made its report in 1973 and recommended that all hospitals offer health education programs to patients and families, both on an inpatient and outpatient basis. The committee also indicated that third-party payment plans should begin paying for such prescribed educational activities. It urged careful evaluation of various educational approaches to determine which ones most improve the patient's health status and reduce the need for health services. It also recommended both preservice and inservice training for health professionals.[20] Committee findings provided a new level of credibility to health education.

The AHA followed the developments of the committee closely and responded to its conclusions. In March 1973 the AHA appointed a Special Committee on Health Education to study the role of hospitals in educating consumers in matters of health, and the role of the AHA in helping hospitals to achieve that objective. The AHA committee concluded:

> Health education is an integral part of high quality health care. Hospitals and other health care institutions, as focal points of community health care, have an obligation to promote, organize, implement, and evaluate health education programs. . . . Through health education programs, hospitals and other health care institutions can contribute to important health care goals, such as improved quality of patient care, better utilization of outpatient facilities, shorter lengths of stay, and reduced health care costs.[21]

In 1973 the AHA also approved "A Patient's Bill of Rights." Six of the twelve sections are related to patient education:

1. Section 2 Information about diagnosis, treatment, and prognosis.
2. Section 3 Procedures determined necessary for the patient's care.
3. Section 7 Need for and alternatives to transfer to other facilities.
4. Section 8 Relationships among those treating the patient.
5. Section 9 Existence of research projects that may affect the patient.
6. Section 10 The patient's requirements for continuing health care following discharge.[22]

The enactment by Congress of the Health Maintenance Organization Act of 1973 represents another progressive step. This legislation requires health maintenance organizations (HMOs) to provide health education for their members.[23] Steps are being taken to implement this requirement, and, as a result, patient education programs are being developed in HMOs all over the country. Several works specific to this topic have been published. (Two of the more significant ones are listed in References at the end of this chapter.)

Focus on Funding

Both the President's Committee on Health Education and the AHA's Special Committee on Health Education indicated that a significant financial commitment was necessary to establish the recommended programs. Both committees concluded that insurance companies had to become involved if the programs were to be implemented. Partially in response to the recommendations of these two committees, the Committee on Health Education of the Health Insurance Benefits Advisory Council issued a report stating that the general thrust of a national health education policy should center on (1) establishment of demonstration projects in settings where meaningful evaluation can be carried out and (2) establishment of training programs designed to improve the quality and quantity of personnel available. The health insurance committee went on to quote from the recommendations of the President's Committee, which stated that the insurance companies should "be willing to adjust premium rates to include in their payments the cost of health education to the patient involved" and "strongly urged private carriers to implement these recommendations as soon as possible."[24]

On another front, the federal Medicare Program also moved to provide coverage for the costs of health education. Since 1974 the Medicare Guidelines for Reimbursement of Patient Education has included coverage for patient education activities considered integral to other covered services. For example, under these guidelines educational activities carried out by nurses, such as, teaching patients to give themselves injections, follow prescribed diets, administer colostomy care, administer medical gases, and carry out other inpatient care activities are often reimbursable as a part of covered routine nursing care. Similarly, the instruction of a patient in the performance of a maintenance program designed by a physical therapist also is often covered. However, when the educational activities are not closely related to the care and treatment of the patient, such as, programs directed toward instructing patients or the general public in preventive health care activities, reimbursement cannot be made. Thus, another segment of society, the federal government, has moved cautiously to endorse the concept of patient education.

ENDORSEMENTS FOR PATIENT EDUCATION

In June 1975 the American Medical Association (AMA) adopted a position paper endorsing organized instruction. The AMA recognized that education of the patient has always been a concern of the physician, but:

> There is a need for a structured educational effort beyond that which the individual member of the team can provide. It is in these situations that planned, patient education programs may be expected to serve. The provision of patient education services designed to assist the patient and his family in the effective management of individual health is a shared and continuous responsibility of both the physician and the patient.[25]

The policy statement went on to detail what an acceptable patient education program should entail.

> Planned patient education programs should be based on identified objectives, should make use of sound educational methods, should have approved content that is scientifically accurate and should be adaptable to the needs of patients. Objectives need to be clarified at the onset along with specific criteria for measuring their achievement. The success or failure of the program should be determined by how well the objectives are realized.[26]

Such farsighted recognition of the potential of patient education has been of great significance in influencing programming. Supportive physicians help convert other hospital personnel.

Another prestigious group soon thereafter also endorsed patient education programming—the Health Insurance Association of America. In a policy statement the association maintained:

> Health Education is the means by which illness and disability can best be prevented, or its impact minimized. . . . A well informed and motivated patient stands a far better chance of an early recovery and is less likely to suffer a recurrence of ill health. This can lead to reduced hospital utilization rates and hence lower costs.[27]

The position paper cited several studies documenting the cost-effectiveness of such programs. One study cited stated that "for every dollar spent for the educational services, $6.00 of medical care costs were saved."[28]

The insurance industry had two principal concerns. One centered on the issues of quality control, standards of practice, and monitoring. Carriers remarked that programs varied widely in effectiveness and stated that a means needed to be developed to reimburse only programs meeting at least minimal standards of practice. The other issue concerned payment for the program. Industry representatives believed that coverage should be "purchased" or paid for by those receiving the services.

The Joint Commission on Accreditation of Hospitals (JCAH) outlined criteria for implementation of patient education.[29]

> The JCAH guidelines specify that educational criteria should be established and approved by the respective professional groups within a hospital and specifically require evidence that the patient has learned (demonstrated knowledge). . . . This section also suggests an interdisciplinary approach to patient education to ensure that patient education efforts are comprehensive and not fragmented.[30]

The AHA approved a policy statement on health promotion in 1979. They defined health promotion to include health information and health education and, as in earlier definitions of health education, stressed informed choice:

> The hospital is identified by the public as the center for health, and thus is looked to as the logical source for all types of information relating to health as well as sickness. It is to the hospital's advantage to encourage this positive image through management support and board-level policy. Further, people look to health professionals as exemplars or models to be copied. Thus, hospitals should take a leadership role in providing appropriate health information and education to their communities, and to the employees of the institution.[31]

The updated policy statement reiterated previous positions taken on health education, but gave additional emphasis to health education programs for hospital employees. Programs were developing in many hospitals that encouraged high-level wellness through exercise, nutrition, stress management, and stop smoking programs. The AHA encouraged and supported such programs as central to the mission of hospitals.

CONCLUSION

The concept of hospital health education has been evolving for more than 25 years. Its remaining obstacle is financial. The acceptance of health education as an integral part of health care is not yet complete. Though encouraged by representatives of health care professions, health care institutions, foundations, accrediting bodies, legislative bodies, a presidential committee, and public demand, it has also been deterred by social, political, and economic conditions. Nevertheless, the prospects for further implementation of health education programs in hospitals appear to be excellent.

NOTES

1. Anne R. Sommers, *Promoting Health* (Germantown, Md.: Aspen Systems Corp., 1976), p. 2.
2. "U.S. Fats and Oils Statistics, 1961–76," *Statistics Bulletin* No. 574 (Washington, D.C.: Economic Research Service, 1977), p. 80.
3. *United States Department of Agricultural Statistics* (Washington, D.C.: US Government Printing Office, 1977).
4. Scott K. Simonds, *Patient Education as One Criteria for Quality Care,* mimeographed (Ann Arbor: Fifth Annual Interdisciplinary Conference on Health Records, 1974), p. 4.
5. S. G. Rosenberg, "Patient Education Leads to Better Care for Heart Patients," *HSMHA Health Reports,* September 1971, pp. 793–802.
6. *Hospital Inpatient Education: Survey Findings and Analyses* (Chicago: American Hospital Association, 1980), p. 42.
7. G. E. Beauchamp, "Patient Education and the Hospital Program," *Veterans Administration Technical Bulletin,* 1953, p. 88.
8. A. M. Johnson et al., "Health Education in Hospitals," *Health Education Journal,* October 1952, pp. 175–185.
9. L. E. Brownell, "Progress in Patient Education," *Health Education at Work,* May 1957.
10. J. Burden, "Doctor Means Teacher," *International Journal of Health Education,* January 1968, pp. 4–12.
11. George Rosen, "Health Education and Preventive Medicine, New Horizons in Medical Care," *American Journal of Public Health,* June 1952, pp. 687–693.
12. H. F. Dowling et al., "Time Spent by Internists on Adult Health Education and Preventive Medicine," *Journal of the American Medical Association,* June 1952, p. 628.
13. Irving Shapiro, *The Patient and Control of Quality in Medical Care. Proceedings Tenth Annual Group Health Institute* (Chicago: Group Health Association of America, 1960).
14. "Health Education in a Hospital Setting," *Currents in Hospital Administration,* August 1962, p. 4.
15. *Health Education in the Hospital, Proceedings of the May 4–5, 1964 AHA Conference* (Chicago: American Hospital Association, 1965), p. 74.
16. Esther Brown, *Newer Dimensions of Patient Care* (New York: Russell Sage Foundation, 1965).

17. *A Model for Planning Patient Education: An Essential Compound of Health Care* (New York: American Public Health Association, 1968), p. 3.
18. Ibid., pp. 9–24.
19. "Review of Research and Studies Related to Patient Education," *Health Education Monograph,* No. 26, 1968, p. 64.
20. Victor Weingarten, "Report of the Findings and Recommendations of the President's Committee on Health Education," *Health Education Monograph,* No. 1, 1974, pp. 11–19.
21. *The Role of Hospitals and Other Health Care Institutions in Personal and Community Health Education* (Chicago: American Hospital Association, 1974), p. 1.
22. *Professional, Accreditation, and Legal Statements Supporting Patient Education* (Chicago: American Hospital Association, 1977), p. 9.
23. Health Maintenance Organization Act of 1973, Title XPII. Sec. 1301, 9.
24. *Report of Committee on Health Education to Health Insurance Benefits Council* 1974, Mimeo, p. 1.
25. *Statement on Patient Education* (Chicago: American Medical Association, June 1975), p. 1.
26. Ibid., p. 2.
27. *Financing In-Hospital Patient Education* (New York: Health Insurance Association of America, 1977), p. 1.
28. Ibid., p. 3.
29. *Accreditation Manual for Hospitals* (Chicago: Joint Commission on Accreditation of Hospitals, 1976).
30. *Professional Accreditation and Legal Statements Supporting Patient Education,* p. 3.
31. *The American Hospital Association's Policy and Statement on the Hospital's Responsibility for Health Promotion* (Chicago: American Hospital Association, 1979).

REFERENCES

Breckon, Donald J. "Highlights in the Evolution of Hospital-Based Patient Education." *Journal of Allied Health,* Summer 1976, pp. 35–39.

Professional, Accreditation, and Legal Statements Supporting Patient Education. Chicago: American Hospital Association, 1977.

Planning Health Education in Health Maintenance Organizations. Washington, D.C.: US Department of Health Education and Welfare, 1976.

A Summary of A Survey of HMO Health Education Programs in the United States. New York: Metropolitan Life Insurance, 1980.

Chapter 2

Hospital Health Education: Nature and Rationale

2

INTRODUCTION

A concept evolving simultaneously in many different places, over a span of more than 25 years is going to bear varying names. So it is with health education. Even in scientific fields, the same term is used by different professionals to convey very different meanings, while, on the other hand, more than one term is used to refer to similar concepts. This lack of precision can cause misunderstanding and confusion. It is particularly important in an emerging discipline to standardize use of terminology. This chapter will attempt to clarify terms used throughout the work in describing hospital health education programs and will present a rationale for such programs.

PROGRAM CHARACTERISTICS

Starting with the most critical, *health education* is an educationally-oriented process of planned change which focuses on those behaviors or problems that directly or indirectly affect people's health.[1] It is sometimes called *hospital or clinical health education* depending on the setting, similar to the differentiation between school or public health education. This use of terminology also helps distinguish such programs from the routine educational endeavors of doctors and nurses, serving to eliminate exclusive ownership of patient education by the medical and nursing professions.

Hospital health education, then, refers to any hospital-based, educationally-oriented process of planned change which focuses on health or illness behaviors, including programs for patients, their families, staff, or members of the general community. *Patient education* involves provision of health education experiences specifically for those who come to health care settings for either inpatient or outpatient care, and usually includes programs for families of patients. In a more narrow sense, *patient teaching* refers specifically to the process of providing health information to patients. Hospital health education is also sometimes called *consumer health education* to distinguish it from hospital inservice or continuing education aimed at staff. *Inservice education* refers to the continuing education activities for hospital staff members seeking to improve their ability to perform job-related tasks. The field often is also referred to as *staff development,* though a slightly larger focus than inservice education is implied. Hospital employees may participate in both inservice education and health education programs.

Health education programs are often provided for staff with the aim of improving their health and, through the role model concept, improving the health of patients. Wellness programs and health promotion programs for hospital employees and their families, for example, are becoming increasingly popular.

The term *health education program* includes all the above, but indicates more than just a collection of isolated educational activities. A program requires comprehensive planning including assessment of both institutional and individual patient needs. A successful program requires that an attempt be made to meet the educational needs of all prospective clients, not just those sufficiently motivated to initiate an educational encounter. A comprehensive program offers carefully planned and evaluated educational activities, employing instructors adequately trained in educational processes.

Families and Outpatients

As noted, a comprehensive program also involves provisions to include family members. Making educational programs available for families is sometimes imperative and always important. Certainly the relatives who must care for a geriatric or pediatric case must understand requirements of treatment. However, those who cook the meals for a male cardiac patient who must undertake a low cholesterol diet also need to fully understand his needs and restrictions. Similarly, family or friends responsible for care of a diabetic, patients on low sodium or sodium-free diets, or anyone on a weight reduction program must also be instructed about proper regimen.

The family member who undertakes an educational program with the patient and staff member is more likely to be supportive of the treatment efforts, and provide reinforcement and encouragement when needed. Compliance with ordered regimens is enhanced when a family member thoroughly understands what is needed and why that regimen is important.

Some health education programs also serve outpatients and their families. There is a great need for expansion of such programming. Consider, for example, the many diabetics diagnosed in a physician's office whose disease has not progressed to the point necessitating hospital admission. They, too, demand education about medicine, diet, exchange lists, lab tests, insulin shock, and diabetic coma. In view of efforts to contain the rising cost of health care by shortening duration of hospital stay, there often is not adequate time for health education. Health education programs need to be added to the list of available outpatient services.

Few programs serve only outpatients. When educational activities exclusively serve outpatients, they are often cosponsored by local health departments and one or more voluntary health agencies. In addition, some doctors' offices employ patient education specialists. They provide services equivalent to those of an outpatient program.

Community Involvement

Many hospitals are increasing their commitment to *community health education* programs, hospital-based educational offerings that "help consumers not only recognize and cope with medical problems, but also prevent them."[2] (This topic is considered in more detail in Chapter 9.) Many hospitals currently provide health education, health maintenance, and health promotion programs for the community. These programs may include, but not be limited to, cardiopulmonary resuscitation techniques, health risk appraisal programs, or risk reduction programs, such as smoking withdrawal and weight control programs. Community health education programs are conducted through radio, television, and newspaper reports, while also using forums such as health fairs, screening programs, and health career days. Program planners often work with the community health agencies in developing and coordinating services. An AHA position paper states:

> Hospitals and other health care institutions, as focal points of community health care, have an obligation to promote, organize, implement, and evaluate health education programs. As a part of this process, hospitals should plan with other health care institutions and community agencies to define each organization's role and responsibility in meeting the health education needs of the populations they serve. . . . Health education that is designed to maintain the good health of the community at large and to prevent illness should be viewed as a service to the community.

> Such services are legitimate activities for hospitals and other health care institutions.[3]

Larger, older hospital-based programs typically serve both inpatients and outpatients, addressing service needs of families of patients, and the community at large. In contrast, newer programs are often exclusively for inpatients and their families.

JUSTIFICATION FOR PROGRAMMING

Regardless of their clientele, hospital health education programs share rationales for beginning service and goals. First, programs should be in the best interests of their patients. Second, patients appreciate individual attention and the opportunities to have their concerns addressed. Finally, as the level of health education increases, patient prognosis often improves.

Hospital care is depersonalized to varying degrees. Patient privacy is sacrificed, along with a degree of dignity. After street clothes are taken, patients are provided a type of uniform, a hospital gown and identification bracelet. Their freedom of movement is restricted as they are surrounded by professionals, mostly in white uniforms, with highly technical, shared jargon. Further, the patient is submitted to extensive testing with intimidating equipment. Most patients are relieved to leave such a place and regain their sense of individuality. Though hospital staff can do much on their own to alleviate these conditions, and often do, patient education programs provide a formal means to address patient fears.

Patient Compliance

As indicated in Chapter 1, patients who fully understand what the physician requests and why that response is important are more likely to comply. Achieving increased compliance is a major reason to initiate educational programs, one that is especially attractive to the medical community. However, achieving higher compliance rates is often difficult. As noted earlier, reinforcement by family members is of utmost importance. Without support from loved ones, the failure of patients to follow ordered weight control programs or smoking withdrawal programs is commonplace. Many patients are not willing or able to comply with a physician's orders, merely because a doctor told them to do so. Extensive individualized instruction may be required to ensure compliance, offering a supplementary group experience with others with similar disorders. Former patients who have regained their health can also be a valuable resource in such programs, as in the American Cancer Society's "Reach To Recovery Program" for mastectomy patients. Individual physicians cannot be expected to provide these time-consuming programs. However, through patient education programming, hospitals can provide such services and are moving to meet such needs.

Increasing patient compliance is not a major goal of some health education programs, especially those which emphasize self-care. Such programs instead prefer the locus of control to center on the individual. Philosophically, these programs prefer to increase personal responsibility and choice. Such an approach avoids blaming the patient for ignorance or noncompliance, instead striving to teach patients to monitor themselves and choose services selectively. (Self-care programs are the focus of Chapter 8.)

Malpractice Suits

Patient education also has the potential of reducing malpractice suits. If it can be established that hospitals or medical staff did not detail to patients what they were consenting to, liability may be established. The emphasis in "informed consent" has shifted from merely giving consent to being adequately informed of the risks involved. The patient's "right to know" has been established in the courts. Accordingly, patient education programs are documenting their efforts, describing what was taught, when, and by whom, as available evidence in the instance of court proceedings.

Furthermore, systems evaluating whether learning has taken place are being used with appropriate documentation. Such efforts have two direct results. Many patients will have no need to file a lawsuit if they have been treated in an open, honest, and humane manner. Second, however, evidence will be available to courts that the patient was taught and that comprehension was demonstrated.

Malpractice suits will never be eliminated. However, good patient education programs may reduce their numbers by paying more attention to the unique needs and interests of the patient.

Health Care Costs

As noted in Chapter 1, HMOs and prepaid plans like Group Health Cooperative and the Kaiser Permanente Plan have demonstrated the cost-saving impact of education programs. Any system of national health insurance Congress may enact would benefit from a strong patient education component. When any entity—a small carrier or the federal government—makes a commitment to pay for the total health care costs of a large number of people, it becomes evident that it is cost-efficient to prevent as many diseases and disorders as possible. Programs directed toward preventing admission or readmission will be viewed favorably in planning a health care plan.

There is also adequate rationale for providing health education programs for employees and their families. When staff members stay healthy, less sick leave and overtime are consumed. Such savings have been used to support industrial safety programs in the past. On-the-job safety programs in industry have expanded to off-the-job programs as well, because sick leave and overtime have to be paid regardless of where the accident occurred. An expansion of this coverage has led many industrial programs to enlarge the scope of their programs from safety to comprehensive health programming, including screening, health education, and other preventive services. The same rationale applies to the provision of programs for hospital staff, which, when added to the "role model" effect on patients as described earlier, further strengthens the case for inhospital health education programs.

The rationale for community health education programs centers on prevention, public service, and public relations. Hospitals have an opportunity to perform a significant and needed public service at relatively low expense, and to gain considerable good will as a result. Such good will can be converted into dollars through wills, gifts, and grants.

There is, then, an extensive, well-developed rationale for hospital health education programming. The patients will be most interested in the individual attention that, in addition to providing answers to specific concerns, reaffirms their sense of individuality. Staff will appreciate the opportunity to improve their own health. The hospital administrator will find most appealing the fact that health education is a good public relations tool. In addition, administration will appreciate being in compliance with recommendations of the AHA, the AMA, the JCAH, and other progressive bodies. Medical staff will find appealing the fact that health education can help reduce malpractice, and that programs will increase patient compliance. Insurance companies and other third party payers will appreciate the potential to reduce health care cost. Finally, all such groups will appreciate the positive effect health education has on health and well-being.

CONCLUSION

Hospital health education programs are here to stay: these programs are needed, wanted, and working. However, standards of practice and funding mechanisms must still be established. Moreover, successful programs must be duplicated in order to increase accessibility and, ultimately, the health status of all involved.

NOTES

1. Helen Ross and Paul Mico, *Theory and Practice in Health Education* (Palo Alto: Mayfield Publishing Co., 1980), p. 7.
2. Peter M. Lazes, ed., *The Handbook of Health Education* (Rockville, Md.: Aspen Systems Corporation, 1979), p. 18.
3. *Statement on the Role and Responsibilities of Hospitals and Other Health Care Institutions in Personal and Community Health Education* (Chicago: American Hospital Association, 1974), p. 2.

REFERENCES

Hospital Inpatient Education: Survey Findings and Analyses. Chicago: American Hospital Association, 1980.

Sommers, Anne, ed. *Health Promotion and Consumer Health Education.* New York: Prodist, 1976.

Part II

Hospital Health Education Programming

part II

Programs develop within institutions in a variety of ways. Usually, they exist because one influential staff member perceived a need or an opportunity and then worked to develop this idea. On the other hand, sometimes programs are developed at the institutional level through work of a committee or department.

More frequently, programs begin with regular patient teaching in one unit within a health care institution. Such programs are often developed intuitively, and the procedures are unique to that institution. On occasion, program developers are not even sure of their actions or the history of their program; ideas evolved with actions deriving from many sources. Such programs and procedures are often difficult to replicate in other institutions because the personnel and circumstances are different. Procedures as well as programs must suit the institution.

Yet some procedures are generally more efficient and effective than others. Program planners can learn from the experiences of others so that they do not have to "reinvent the wheel." Existent programs might have been improved if better planning had taken place. Failed programs might have succeeded if implemented differently.

Part II discusses in "cookbook style" some successful procedures for planning, implementing, administering, and evaluating a hospital health education program. It is intentionally basic and general, so as to be most useful for planners considering initiation of a health education program. Those with responsibility for hospital health education should select strategies which will be most useful in their institutions. Institutional, management, health service, client, resource, and programmatic characteristics are all factors that affect planning, implementing, and evaluating procedures.[1] The principles and procedures discussed in this section can be successfully applied to a large variety of hospitals and medical care settings.

NOTE

1. *A Model for Patient Education Programming.* (Washington, D.C.: American Public Health Association, 1979), p. 4.

Chapter 3

Planning a Health Education Program

3

INTRODUCTION

There is no single agreed upon way to effectively plan and initiate a health education program. Variations occur that depend on the hospital involved, its administrative patterns, past experience with health education, clientele, and the experience, values, and attitudes of hospital staff regarding such programs. There are, however, some procedures that have worked for other facilities that should be reviewed for use by program developers. This chapter explores procedures used by practitioners in developing successful health education programs.

ASSESSING THE STATUS OF HEALTH EDUCATION

An important initial step of program development is to determine "what was" and "what is" before developing "what will be." There is a tendency on the part of program developers to assume that they are starting at the outset, often to the amusement or chagrin of those aware of past attempts to develop similar programs. Assessing the status of ongoing health education will provide a basis for proposed programs. It also helps stimulate early support for programs by associating proposals with a variety of people.

There is an old adage useful in planning and initiating a program: "There is no limit to what can be accomplished if you don't care who gets the credit." Discovering who has developed health education programs in the past and who is currently involved in such projects, and building on these efforts, is frequently critical to the success of a program proposal, generating support from those who have been given credit, and minimizing resistance from those who know that their colleagues are already involved in health education efforts. Giving credit to those contributing to past and current efforts can help develop credibility and support, both of which are essential to hospital health educators as pioneers in a new field.

Gathering Information

One place to begin in collecting data is with long-term employees. Hospital administrators, administrative secretaries, nursing directors, inservice directors, unit supervisors, and other key personnel who have been with the institution for a long period of time can be a valuable source of information. Lunch or a coffee break is an especially good time to get them talking about past or present health education activities. Casual conversation is also a good means to securing a feeling for potential support or resistance to programs.

Annual reports, mission statements, policies, and other written records may reveal past practices and commitments. These documents may be located in a variety of places depending on the hospital. A few apt questions will usually determine their existence and location, so they can be located and reviewed at least briefly. It is important to know what has been officially stated and what has been omitted.

Program planners also should contact administrative personnel at various levels of responsibility, whether or not of long-time service to the institution. Such people often are "gatekeepers" of necessary documents. It is also critical for administrators to know what is being done and why in order to educate them about hospital health education. The occasions can be used to discuss activities outside one's own hospital. Administrators should be sent copies of appropriate articles or program descriptions, usually resulting in continued support and confidence. Asking for advice and assistance and following through on suggestions can provide enormous dividends. Again, in talking and writing about health education, others should be credited for their suggestions and help.

Other valuable techniques include using the staff newsletter or posting a notice on prominent bulletin boards. A brief description of needed assistance will frequently stimulate people to volunteer information that might not otherwise have been shared. In addition, public notice keeps the concept of health education in the minds of the staff, regardless of whether it spurs immediate involvement. Behavioral theorists suggest that such awareness is the necessary first step in spawning interest and support for an idea.

Formal Survey

In larger hospitals it is usually necessary to perform a formal staff survey to secure an accurate picture of the status of health education efforts.

Formal surveys are preferable in smaller hospitals as well. Planned, formal surveys enhance the accuracy of the assessment by ensuring breadth and consistency of questioning. Exhibit 3-1 presents a general guide to survey preparation and presentation.

A single staff survey may have several purposes and formats. An important and often overlooked initial step is to clearly state in writing the purpose of the survey, vital in determining the format and the content of the survey.

Useful surveys can focus on past or present health education programs, on the need for patient education as perceived by the hospital staff, or on the interest of staff members in health education. Though there may be more than one reason for conducting the survey, it is preferable to combine information gathering from the staff at large into one approach, rather than contacting them on several separate occasions, that is, unless the requests are a year or more apart.

A second and equally important step is to identify precisely the survey universe. Knowing the purpose of the survey and who will be questioned are basic to the format and content of the effort.

The format will vary depending on the size of the hospital, the time available for information gathering, and the objectives of the survey planners. If the purpose is to retrieve a relatively small amount of information from a large number of people, a questionnaire is the preferred format, as shown in Exhibit 3-2. On the other hand, if the purpose is to secure a large amount of information from a small number of people, an interview is preferred. Interviews are more effective than written surveys in assessing the direction and intensity of feelings and attitudes of the subject.

Developing and using either questionnaires or interviews is complex. Suggested readings at the end of the chapter further discuss these simple guidelines which hospital personnel should follow in order to plan and conduct successful surveys.

DESIGNING THE PLANNING PROCESS

The effectiveness of planning processes varies with the settings, the people involved, the resources available, the amount of administrative support and the time frame available to perform the planning. One constant, however, remains; the most effective process is itself preplanned by the person or persons with the responsibility to coordinate the planning. Good planning just doesn't happen by itself.

The staff member planning and initiating a hospital health education program must firstly have a clear vision of what is being proposed, resulting

Exhibit 3–1 Tips on Performing Surveys

General

1. Carefully state in writing the purpose of the survey.
2. Decide precisely what individuals and groups will be surveyed.
3. Determine what administrative approval, if any, is needed for performing the survey and obtain authorization.
4. Develop a draft of the questionnaire or interview schedule. Ask only questions directly related to the written purpose or restating the purpose of the survey.
5. Ask three to six people to serve as a "jury of experts" by reviewing the instrument and suggesting improvement. Revise accordingly.
6. Conduct a pilot study by surveying a small portion of the survey universe; or by performing a "practice run" on a group similar to those to be surveyed. Revise as needed.
7. Prepare final copies of the questionnaire or interview schedule. Be sure that the survey instrument is brief, well-organized, and professional in appearance.
8. Consider using the staff newsletter to describe the survey and solicit cooperation, and a subsequent issue to announce the results.

Questionnaires

1. Prepare an attractive cover letter that clearly states what information is sought and why that information is important. Indicate administrative support for the survey. Sign each copy, preferably in a bright blue ink.
2. Consider the advantages and disadvantages of anonymity of those questioned and decide upon an approach.
3. If feasible, distribute the questionnaire at staff meetings when participants can complete entire survey.

Interviews

1. Set up an appointment for the interview to be free from interruptions for 15 to 30 minutes.
2. Introduce yourself and the survey. Try to establish rapport by making the respondent feel comfortable and at ease. Express self-confidence through voice, comments, facial expressions, and eye contact. Act interested in the responses.

Exhibit 3–1 continued

4. If hospital mail is used, specify a return date of one week. Supply return information at bottom of each questionnaire.
5. If survey is not anonymous, send follow-up note and, if possible, another questionnaire to nonrespondents. (Final response rates vary from 15 to 85%, depending on effectiveness of presentation, ease of response, and interest of the respondents in the survey topic.)
6. If department heads are asked to distribute and collect the questionnaires, contact them personally at regular intervals to be sure the questionnaires have actually reached potential respondents.

3. Be familiar enough with the interview schedule to try to adhere to it without being unduly constrained. Keep minimal notes, but immediately after the interview write a more elaborate summary of the interview.
4. Listen actively. Observe tone and volume of voice, pace of speech, and gestures. Such behaviors are often the clues to the individual's true feelings.
5. Probe gently! Wait for answers, clarify without leading the interviewee. Paraphrase or repeat questions as needed.
6. Conduct the interview at an appropriate pace. Summarize the interview or in other ways bring it to a natural conclusion. Thank the interviewee.

from familiarity with the literature, visits to existing programs, and discourse with colleagues at professional meetings. Such a vision gives purpose and direction to the planning initiative while providing a sense of confidence and hope to the planning team.

Resources

Budgeted funds should be available for purchasing material, visiting other programs, attending professional conferences, and employing consultants, along with resources providing for normal secretarial support services. The amount of planning dollars necessary will vary with the staff, background and the health care facility. There already may be a travel budget alloted for the educational staff. The hospital staff may routinely attend conferences; a library budget may already be supplied or most of the relevant books and journals already may have been purchased by the hospital. The planners already may be familiar with existing health edu-

Exhibit 3–2 Sample Hospital Staff Survey to Assess the Status of Health Education

The Education Department, with the approval and support of central administration, would like to determine (1) what health education activities have been or are being conducted in this hospital, (2) if the staff members feel that there is a need for an expanded hospital health education program, and (3) the amount of interest in such a program. Department heads and other key people in the hospital are accordingly being asked to complete this brief questionnaire which should take only five minutes to complete. Please return to the Education Department by this Friday.

Name________________ Position____________ Unit________

__ Yes __ No Has your unit or does your unit routinely conduct any formally planned health education activities for patients, their families, unit staff, or the community at large? If yes, please specify.

Target Group	Educational Activity	Contact Person
1.		
2.		
3.		

__ Yes __ No Do you or your staff spend a significant amount of time conducting informal health education, such as, answering questions and explaining procedures? Please estimate the percentage of staff time spent.

__ 0 to 10% __ 25 to 50%
__ 10 to 25% __ 50 to 75%

__ Yes __ No Do you feel that patients leaving your unit adequately understand their condition and have adequate knowledge for self-care after discharge? Please estimate the percentage of patients who have such knowledge.

__ 0 to 10% __ 50 to 75%
__ 10 to 25% __ 75 to 100%
__ 25 to 50%

__ Yes __ No Do you feel that family members responsible for patient care adequately understand the patient's condition and needed care?

__ Yes __ No Do you feel that patients and families desire more health education than they are currently receiving in your unit?

Exhibit 3–2 continued

___ Yes ___ No Do you feel that you and the majority of your staff are adequately trained to provide health education for the patients, their families, and the community at large?

___ Yes ___ No Do you feel that you and your staff possess adequate time to meet the health education service needs of your unit?

___ Yes ___ No Would you like to see the Education Department conduct inservice sessions to assist you and your staff in improving your health education skills?

___ Yes ___ No Would you like to see the Education Department expand its services and offer health education activities to ___ your patients, ___ their families, ___ your staff, ___ the community at large?

Thank you for your time and interest. Again, please return the completed questionnaire to the Education Department by this Friday.

cation programs. Consultation may be available without charge from nearby colleges or universities. Upper-level students may even be available to serve as planning staff assistants to earn educational credit.

Another important consideration during the planning stage is the assembly of needed materials. Planners should organize a readily accessible file of position papers and other supportive papers. Appropriate books and journals should be ordered. Drug retail personnel and other product sales representatives should be contacted for educational material. A standing request to the purchasing department to have sales representatives contact the education department is usually sufficient, though it is also appropriate to communicate directly with the company's national office. Chapter 7 lists names and addresses of major pharmaceutical companies. A file should be assembled of representative materials.

Timetable

The planners need to agree on the timetable for their efforts. Indeed, many good planners use variations of the Program Evaluation and Review Techniques (PERT).[1] To use PERT, it is necessary to briefly state the goal of the planning process and then to list in sequence all the steps or activities needed to accomplish that result. A target date is established for program implementation and a timetable developed for each phase of the process. The PERT process also recommends diagramming so that planners can tell quickly at what stage of the process they are and whether or not they are on schedule. Exhibit 3-3 illustrates a typical PERT chart as applied to patient education.

INVOLVEMENT OF OTHERS

With the completion of background work, it is time to involve others in the planning process. Committees usually take longer than an individual to complete a project because of difficulties in organizing and the length of time spent on discussion. Committee participation calls for give and take and the trade-offs may not be mutually acceptable. Most planners know of the oft-repeated adage, "a camel is a horse that was planned by a committee."

Exhibit 3–3 Patient Education PERT Chart

	Tasks	*Date to be Accomplished*
12	Implementation of a postcardiac education program	1-2-83
11	Staff training, internal publicity	12-82
10	Pretest and revise accordingly	11-82
9	Physician review and suggested revision	10-82
8	ICU staff review and subsequent revision	10-82
7	Pharmacy staff review	10-82
6	Respiratory therapy review	10-82
5	Developments of goals and objectives, activities, evaluation, record keeping	9-82
4	Development of patient/family information packet	9-82
3	Visitation of one or more postcardiac education programs	8-82
2	Library research, literature research	8-82
1	Visitation of American Heart Association unit	8-82

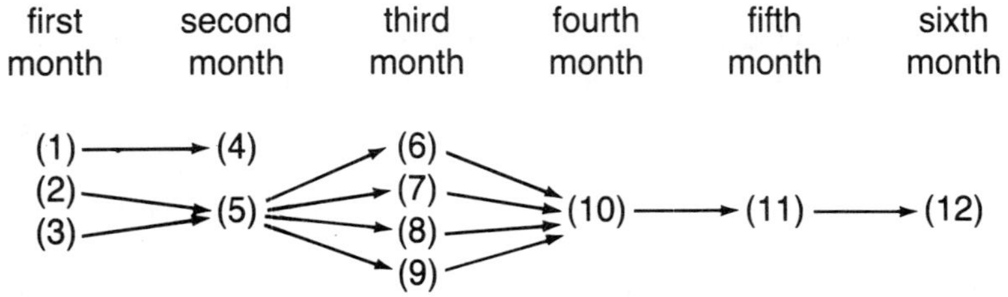

It is vital for at least two reasons to involve a variety of people in planning the program. First, program planners need the insight and understanding that comes from involving representatives from a cross section of hospital units. An insider's understanding of people and programs in the various units is helpful in determining what will work and what will not. Even in a small hospital, no one person enjoys that perspective. Second, and of even more importance, members of the various units need to be involved early in the process so a sense of ownership is established. If personnel feel that the program being developed is their own, a high level of future support and cooperation is likely. Planners can facilitate development of a sense of ownership by well-chosen words in approaching and in working with future members of the planning committee.

Committee Structure

Before appointing a new committee, an analysis should be made of existing ones, with particular attention paid to their charge and membership. A valid complaint is that institutions often have too many committees and that people often resist serving on another. If an existing committee has a charge that encompasses health education, has time to complete the work schedule in the anticipated time frame, and has a chairperson and membership interested in health education, it may be appropriate to use that body to plan the program. Usually, however, it is preferable to establish a new committee with a specific charge and timetable in which to develop the program.

One should decide in advance whether the body is to be *ad hoc* (temporary), or standing. Most often, planning committees have a longevity of one year or less and their contacts differ from those of standing committees. Prospective participants are more willing to accept membership on a committee if the time commitments are clear in advance.

Similarly, the charge to the committee should be written and used in the recruitment process. Appropriate administrative review should be obtained for formation and operation of a committee in order to effectively plan and implement programs.

A list of prospective committee members should be developed. More than one person should assist in developing the list or should review possible choices with the opportunity of suggesting others. Consideration should be given to offering committee membership to professionals key to operating a health education program, such as the director of nursing, a dietician, a physician, a discharge planner or social worker, and the director of public relations. Similarly, those with experience in health education or with a high level of interest and enthusiasm should also be included. Surprisingly, it often works well to also tap for committee membership staff members who are vocal critics of patient education. This criticism is often based on a lack of knowledge and serving on the committee would be educational. It is also reassuring to the hospital community at large to know that all points of view have been considered, though not necessarily incorporated in the proposal. In sum, the committee should be representative, balanced, willing to work, open to other points of view, and appointed with a specific charge to be completed within a specific time frame.

Committees work best with 7 to 12 members, though the size of the hospital will affect the size of the committee. If the committee grows much larger than 12, consideration should be given to formation of an executive or work committee to prepare material for review and comment of the larger group.

A decision should be made before the committee assembles on who will chair the group. Appointment of the chairperson concurrent with the appointment of committee membership ensures that the chair will have the ability, time, and commitment to the task. Strong consideration should be given to appointing a chairperson from the staff of the Education Department.

Appropriate publicity concerning the appointment of the committee should be disseminated within the hospital and among the community media. The media is especially good for enhancing levels of awareness and support.

Working committees usually need time blocks of one and a half to two hours to accomplish work. Meetings should begin and end on schedule and dates for the series of meetings should be announced early, members being requested to keep these dates in mind. A schedule convenient for all is difficult to arrange, but input on the best meeting time should be sought. Those unable to attend meetings should be informed of topics, discussions, and outcomes, and given the opportunity to submit ideas in writing.

CONCLUSION

The tasks of a planning committee will vary. These tasks include recommending policy statements, developing a framework for an institution-wide health education program with a timetable for implementation, and reviewing specific components of the institutional program. These topics will be addressed in Chapter 4.

NOTE

1. Lawrence Green, et al., *Health Education Planning, A Diagnostic Approach* (Palo Alto, California: Mayfield Publishing Company, 1980), p. 119.

REFERENCES

A Model for Patient Education Programming. Washington, D.C.: American Public Health Association, 1979.

Bradburn, Norman. *Improving Interview and Questionnaire Design.* San Francisco: Jossey Bass, 1979.

Dillman, Don. *Mail and Telephone Surveys.* New York: John Wiley and Sons, 1978.

Implementing Patient Education in the Hospital. Chicago: American Hospital Association, 1979. (Chapters 1–6.)

Pritchett, Sue. *Patient, Family and Community Health Education: Design and Management of Hospital Based Programs.* Atlanta: Pritchett & Hull Associates, 1977.

Chapter 4

Relationships with the Board, the Administration, and Other Units

4

INTRODUCTION

Each hospital health education program has characteristics unique to its institution reflecting past practices of the hospital and the personal impact of the program developers. It is important that programs are adapted to the time and place. A program's unique features also help establish a sense of ownership and pride. However, regardless of the setting or the nomenclature, relationships with the board of directors, the administration, and other units need to be clarified.

POLICIES

For any program to succeed, it is important to secure the support of top-level management, including governing boards. Formal approval of policy establishes commitments, and clarifies institutional responsibilities to patients and their families, staff, and the community. Such a policy also helps provide legitimacy and credibility to the program.

Policies serve as a framework within which a program can be developed. A policy statement details the scope of commitment and serves as a guideline for implementation in the various departments. It also represents a continuing reminder to midlevel managers of an institution's commitment to health education.

It is possible for programs to function without a formally approved policy statement. Indeed, a survey conducted by the AHA indicates that such policies are of relatively recent origin. Many hospitals have had in writing only a statement of general philosophy that made a cursory reference to education; others have had informal or unwritten policies, procedures, and philosophies.

Hospital administrators are now recognizing the advantages of clearly stating a policy and of having it formally approved. Confusion among the staff is minimized, commitment to the concept is enhanced, and the public relations value of the policy statement is magnified.

Staff members with responsibility for policy development need to obtain copies of any existing institutional policy statements that encompass or make reference to health education. Similarly, they need to fully understand the process for adoption of new policies and the timetable for such board actions. Procedures usually require administrative willingness to support the new policy and, in most cases, boards of directors are reluctant to approve items the administrator does not support.

Administrative support is more probable if key personnel have been involved in developing or revising the policy document. A common procedure is for a staff member to study existing policy statements and develop a draft that conforms to standard format. The document is then studied and revised by a health education committee and distributed for review among key members of the administrative staff. After consideration of their comments, the document should be revised, this time for clarity and precision, before being presented to the board of directors. Content and format of the policy statement may vary significantly. Exhibit 4–1 provides a sample demonstrating the typical elements to be addressed in a statement of policy.

This sample policy statement assumes that the health education program will be centralized. Smaller hospitals or hospitals with new health education programs are often decentralized with authority for educational programming vested in each unit. This type of system can result in duplication of equipment and, more importantly, significant variation in emphasis and quality between units in a hospital. If, on the other hand, it is not financially feasible to establish an education department, but sufficient interest resides in the appropriate units, a decentralized system can work. The sample policy statement would then need to be rewritten to eliminate or reduce the role of the education department and increase the responsibilities of the various participating units.

STAFF TITLES

The degree of centralization of a hospital's health education program will also have an impact on whether the title director, coordinator, or educator will be used. Choice of title should reflect the institutional position as described in the policy statement. If the program is centralized, that is, a specific person is responsible for health education, the term director of

Exhibit 4–1 Hospital Health Education Policy

Community Hospital endorses the commitment to hospital health education as expressed in the policy statements of the American Hospital Association and as reflected in that body's "A Patient's Bill of Rights." Community Hospital is committed to providing meaningful educational activities to patients and their families, hospital staff, and members of the community designed to enhance self-care, improve health status, and generally promote a high level of wellness.

The responsibility for such educational programming will be diffused throughout the departments and units with an opportunity to provide such education. Responsibility for coordination and supervision will reside in the Department of Education.

The Director of Health Education will assist staff within appropriate units in the development of programs consistent with sound educational practice. These programs will include learner/staff involvement in the assessment of learning needs, selection of preferred learning methods from a variety of plans, and evaluation and documentation of the degree of learning.

Discharge planning shall include a review of the patient's assessed learning needs, a discussion of opportunities offered for outpatients, and a discussion of community agencies offering educational opportunities.

All health education programs will be reviewed by the Health Education Committee and approved by the Director of Health Education.

Community Hospital believes that its staff should, as far as possible, be role models exemplifying good health habits and a high level of wellness. To assist staff in accomplishing this goal, health education programs geared specifically to the health needs of staff will be designed by the Education Department. Again, as with programs for patients and their families, staff opportunities should conform to sound educational practice. Staff members are expected to participate in these activities.

Community Hospital will support and work cooperatively with other community agencies in conducting health education activities aimed at promoting high-level wellness among the residents of the community. Staff and facilities for conducting such activities will be made available if feasible. Community Hospital is committed to serving as a focal point for meeting the health needs of the service population.

health education or some equivalent title should be used which reflects the level of authority. Under such a structure, the director of health education would have authority, responsibility, and, presumably, salary equivalent to the director of nursing and heads of other units.

If the intent of the planners is to have a health education specialist assist the various units and coordinate, though not have authority over their efforts, then the title of health education coordinator or its equivalent is used. The responsibilities of coordinators can vary significantly and should be detailed by the planners. (Job descriptions are discussed in detail in Chapter 5.)

The term patient educator is usually reserved for staff members with responsibilities for patient teaching, but with little or no administrative responsibility. Patient educators may be appointed within units in addition to a director or coordinator, or in lieu of such persons. Again, a clear vision of what best suits the particular institutional setting at a given time must guide such decision making.

PLACEMENT IN THE ORGANIZATIONAL CHART

A related matter requiring an early decision for institutions with a centralized program concerns the placement of the director or coordinator of health education within the institutional authority structure. The existing administrative flow chart should be obtained and studied before making this decision.

Typically, the director or coordinator reports to the hospital administrator, the director of nursing, or the personnel director. There are advantages and disadvantages to having the health education program under any one of these three positions. The choice will no doubt be affected by personalities, as well as administrative philosophy.

Reporting to Administrator

It is preferable for the director of health education to report directly to the administrator of the hospital, in a manner similar to other directors. Such placement makes clear the commitment to education by indicating that the education department is on equal footing with all other departments in the hospital. Meetings of department heads then can serve as forums to discuss programs, problems, or functions that arise between units. Such discourse between department heads or directors in the presence of central administration can be critical to the success of programs, such as health education, that rely on the cooperation of other units.

If the unit reports as other units do, it is assumed that budget-making procedures will also be similar. Health education programs do not necessarily need as large a budget as other units, but they do need access to funds. In decentralized programs, too, the alloted budget should be clearly detailed, even though the program is part of several different budgets. The danger of not having a separate budget principally lies in lack of control: when funds are limited and new funding priorities are set, those controlling the budgets that have funded past health education activities may decide not to fund health education activities any longer. There is considerable truth in the parody of the Golden Rule, "Those that have the gold rule!"

Administrators responsible for a health education program need to have a budget they control. Program directors cannot be reduced to begging or surviving on discretionary funds controlled by others. Such arrangements make programs vulnerable and survival tenuous. Specifics to development of a budget will be discussed in greater detail later in this chapter.

Reporting to Director of Nursing

The health education unit can also report to the director of nursing. The chief advantage of such an arrangement is that nursing staff have a great deal of opportunity and concomitant responsibility to perform health education for patients and their families. Indeed, in some hospitals, all patient education is performed by members of the nursing staff and is viewed as a standard nursing function.

The American Nurses' Association states that:

> Every professional nurse is responsible and accountable to the patient and family for the quality of nursing care the patient receives. This responsibility and accountability includes teaching the patient and family relevant facts about special health care needs and supporting appropriate modification of behavior.[1]

Health education programs do, as previously discussed, have the responsibility of working with units other than nursing. That relationship is not as explicit when the entity is located within the nursing unit. If the director of nursing strongly supports health education and is able to work well with the health education specialist, this arrangement can work well. If, because of personality conflicts or philosophical differences, these conditions are not present, the arrangement can severely limit the effectiveness of a health education program.

A major disadvantage of having the health education program report to the director of nursing relates to the matter of bureaucracy. If all administrative decisions have to first go through the director of nursing, the review would necessarily take longer. More importantly, however, vital items could be filtered or eliminated from the administrator's review. Again, the health education program could become limited.

Unfortunately, there is considerable precedent for controversy to develop between nurses and health educators. Such role conflicts, territoriality, and turf-guarding must be resolved for programs to have their maximum impact. With a tradition of performing health education activities, nurses often feel that it is within their professional right to continue to do so. Many consider health educators deficient in background, training, and experience. Health educators, on the other hand, often feel that nurses have performed little formal health education and what they have done, they have done poorly. The truth is probably somewhere between these two extremes and the best solution is to develop a team approach.

As was noted in Chapter 1, nurses have been involved in health education activities for generations, meeting a critical need. That need has grown and activated consumers are demanding more health education than ever before. Concurrently, other job demands on nurses have increased significantly so, in truth, many nurses do not have time to devote to patient education. Because of consumer demand, health education is rapidly developing in sophistication. Many nurses are not commonly taught to function as education specialists or to apply proper learning theory to endeavors in patient education.

The team approach has evolved from the increased consumer demand for health education, along with the lack of specific training in educational skills at associate degree nursing schools, and the lack of time and interest on the part of many nurses to be responsible for health education. The team approach suggests that doctors, nurses, dieticians, therapists, and technologists are all part of the health care team. All have important information to share with the patient and family or with the community at large. An educational specialist can be added to the team to design and implement programs and coordinate the efforts of team members to meet educational needs. This team philosophy to running a program is presently being adopted in many hospitals.

Reporting to Director of Personnel

Some health education programs report to the director of personnel. This placement often dates from the establishment of an inservice training unit, now called continuing education or staff development.

When health education services are within the purview of personnel, it is important that the relationship to continuing education and staff responsibilities be clarified at the outset. Administrative overhead can be reduced by having one department head supervising the entire education department. When this occurs, however, staff members should have clearly delineated responsibilities. When one person directs all educational responsibilities, patient education and community health education, newer than continuing education, often receive minimal attention. This can be avoided with adequate planning.

The obvious advantage of having education functions combined in a single department such as personnel and supervised by one department head is that coordination of effort, budget, equipment, materials, and personnel can occur more readily. In hospitals where staff development programs are already located in the personnel department and where qualified personnel are heading that unit, an entire educational program may be placed there by expanding the existing program.

Health education programs designed for staff most logically can be placed in personnel. For decentralized programs, additional rationale can be developed for locating patient education functions in personnel because the staff in several units will be performing patient and family education in their own unit. Such placement often does not work as well for more centralized programs and usually does not fix responsibility for community education.

The most desirable situation suggests that a health education unit be created with the director or coordinator reporting directly to the hospital administrator, and being treated as are other directors or department heads. Other arrangements described above may be successful, if personalities involved are willing to make them work. However, there is no single correct answer to where the health education program should be placed.

DEVELOPING THE BUDGET

Planners need to anticipate expenses that the program will incur and develop a budget that will include adequate income for financing those expenses. Budgets are usually annual, with a variety of possible fiscal years used. Necessary background work for the development of a budget involves determining the established fiscal year and obtaining a copy of the institution's budget for the current operating year. It is also appropriate to study the operating budget of major units, such as nursing, in order to discover if funds are currently designated for health education. Another important element is to involve those with budgetary experience. At a minimum, deadlines for submission of a proposal and the amount of required supporting detail should be known. It is also helpful to be aware of who reviews and decides on the proposals, and what reviews or opportunity for revision exist.

When a budget is developed for a new unit, the funds will usually be allocated from the institution's general funds. Later, there may be some income for the health education program from sources such as third party reimbursement or direct billing of patients. These payments will ordinarily be handled by the division that controls all other hospital income. (A more detailed discussion of funding philosophy is found in Chapter 10.)

Obtaining program funding by this procedure is not only fiscally, but also, educationally sound. Programs that generate income may be required to place undue emphasis on raising funds or may be required to be fiscally self-sufficient. Immediate or start-up funds are often large and plateau after a year or two of operation. The long-term impact on health care costs can offset these high start-up costs. Often it is also advisable to develop a budget for the first three years of the program's operation, in order to phase in equipment purchases and staff additions, for instance. Administrators like to see the complete financial plan, not just the first phase.

Budget formats will vary between institutions so planners should work with appropriate members of the administrative staff in developing a sound proposal. While the items may be labeled or grouped differently, budgets routinely include: (1) staff salaries, (2) support staff salaries, (3) educational materials (including pamphlets, posters, and media purchase or rental), (4) equipment purchase or rental and maintenance, (5) staff development (to include travel, conference fees, and tuition costs), (6) purchase of books and subscriptions to journals and newsletters, and (7) other unit operating costs, such as, postage, telephone, photocopying, and refreshments.

A final cautionary note regarding inflation must be added for neophytes to the budget planning process. A budget must provide for actual costs a year in advance, which can amount to 10 to 20 percent in excess of current costs. An estimate of the rate of inflation and its effect on the various categories of costs must be made. Budgets can be strained and programs curtailed because planners fail to account for the inflation factor.

CONCLUSION

Relationships with the board, the administration, and other units must be developed and tended with care if the health education program is to be successful. Such elements are part of a sound foundation on which to build. Administrative support is critical to the success of a new program and is evidenced by placement in the organizational chart, title, authority invested in the program, and involvement in decision making. Educational programs are part of the institution's many services. Efforts must be made to ensure that other units of the institution recognize and support the contributions of education to the mission of the hospital.

NOTE

1. *Standards of Nursing Practice* (Kansas City: American Nurses' Association, 1973).

REFERENCES

American Hospital Association. *Implementing Patient Education in the Hospital.* Chicago: American Hospital Association, 1979. (Chapter 6.)

Pritchett, Sue. *Patient, Family and Community Health Education: Design and Management of Hospital Based Programs.* Atlanta: Pritchett and Hull Associates, 1977. (Pages 10–15.)

Squyres, Wendy D., ed. *Patient Education: An Inquiry into the State of the Art.* New York: Springer Publishing Co., 1980. (Chapter 9.)

Chapter 5

Staff Selection and Training

5

INTRODUCTION

With the planning process underway, and with the support and approval of the various boards and units, attention should be directed to selecting the staff for the program. Participants should be chosen with considerable care. Staff can often break a program, even though the planning stages have gone quite well. It is important that staff be selected from individuals who are truly interested in health education. They should either have specific training for the program or be willing to obtain it. Staff members should also possess the kind of personality that permits them to interact easily with clients.

SELECTING LEADERSHIP AND STAFF MEMBERS

The key to a successful program of hospital health education is selecting a person who can provide the necessary leadership to sell the program to staff, patients, and the community. That kind of leadership suggests commitment, enthusiasm, ability to communicate effectively orally and in writing, and a knowledge-base of necessary actions deriving from training and work experience. If the leadership is to be effective in implementing the program, two other characteristics come into play. First, the director must be astute to the political dimensions of the job and must work effectively with people through formal and informal channels. Second, the manager must be willing to work long and hard, often in the face of adversity, to accomplish the task of building a successful health education program.

Job Description

The initial consideration for selecting leadership is a definition of the job. Agreement should be reached early on a job description that describes both responsibilities and qualifications. The nature of the job description will vary considerably, as discussed earlier, depending on whether a director, coordinator, or patient educator is desired. Exhibit 5–1 provides a sample job description for the position of director.

If a patient educator position is being filled, then education and experience requirements would be considerably less demanding than those for a director. Often, the patient educator is an R.N. with some training or work experience in teaching. Such minimal qualifications can be appropriate if the job is narrowly defined as, for example, in teaching diabetic patients, or if there is adequately trained supervision available.

The patient educator should at least possess a background in both the physical and social sciences and have some course work in human behavior. He or she should have a knowledge of the institution's medical terminology, patient care, and staff roles, and must also be trained in health education methodology. The patient educator must bring to the health care team an expertise that enables him or her to be effective and that inspires confidence among other members of the team. Variations on the title, patient educator, include: (1) clinical health educator, (2) health educator, and (3) health education specialist.

Internal or External Search

An early consideration in selecting leadership involves the decision whether to restrict the search for personnel to candidates within the institution or to conduct an external search. Either process is acceptable, if it results in good leadership. Advantages and disadvantages to both approaches ought to be considered before a decision is made.

It is fairly typical to select a patient educator from within. When this occurs, he or she is often an RN with special interests, natural abilities, and training specific to the job. It is less common to select a coordinator or director from within the health care facility, unless the hospital has a large staff of educational specialists from which to select. When an internal candidate is selected without the necessary training or work experience, the effectiveness of the program is compromised at the outset. Simply adding the duties of directing a health education program to the job description of an existing staff member should be avoided. In such cases, staffers usually do not have the training, work experience, or time to devote to the additional tasks, and often lack interest and enthusiasm in the program. Busy staff members are likely to concentrate on their traditional responsibilities and direct only a token effort to the health education program.

Exhibit 5–1 Director of Hospital Health Education

A. Responsibilities

1. Manages the activities of the Health Education Department, supervises secretarial staff, and responds to all central administration requests.
2. Reviews all existing health education programs, and works with the appropriate personnel to improve and standardize offerings.
3. Reviews and approves all proposals for new health education programs, and ensures that such proposals have also been reviewed by appropriate personnel.
4. Consults with personnel in various departments, and assists them in planning, implementing, and evaluating new or continuing patient education programs.
5. Coordinates interdepartmental health education programs.
6. Approves purchase of educational materials and equipment; coordinates use of same among departments.
7. Maintains and disseminates current literature and other material regarding patient education theory, methodology, and media use.
8. Solicits internal and external sources of support for health education; manages expenditure of same.
9. Coordinates interdepartmental committees, and assists departmental committees concerned with health education.
10. Maintains contact with related community health agencies.

B. Desirable skills and competencies

1. Ability to communicate effectively both orally and in writing. Projects a positive image.
2. Knowledge of the decision-making structure and how it operates with the ability to work effectively within that structure.
3. Knowledge of group dynamics. Ability to work effectively with committees in leadership and membership roles.
4. Ability to develop program plans with goals, objectives, implementation, and evaluation components.
5. Knowledge of educational methodologies, media, and materials. Ability to teach effectively.
6. Creativity, receptiveness to input from many sources.
7. Problem solving talents. Ability to analyze, solicit needed data, synthesize, compromise, and develop a workable solution to problems.
8. Professional initiative and assertiveness resulting in completion of needed tasks.

Exhibit 5–1 continued

C. Requirements
1. Master's Degree in Health Education with appropriate course work or work experience in hospital health education, plus two years of related work experience, or
2. Bachelor's Degree in Health Education, plus three years experience in hospital-based health education programs.

Again, as indicated earlier, the commitment of central administration is important and should be cultivated. Some administrators simply add health education responsibilities to an already overworked staff member without expecting much output, in order to possess on paper a program they can point to when it is politically appropriate. Committed administrators, on the other hand, will hire trained and experienced personnel, provide a sufficient budget and authority-base from which to operate, and demand accountability in the form of a well-developed and well-run program.

Staff Size

The number of staff selected and trained depends on the size of the institution, and the type and size of the program. Institutional size is not necessarily the biggest variable. Small institutions may have a number of programs that serve almost all of their staff and patients, and are made available to families and outpatients. They may also have a large-scale community health education program. On the other hand, large institutions may not offer staff programs or services for families and outpatients, and health education may only be available for patients in one or two units. Again, the number of staff selected and trained will depend upon the commitment to health education and the number of clients to be served.

The number of staff will also depend upon whether the program is centralized or decentralized. If the program is centralized, the health education staff will be comparatively smaller, and will, ideally, be trained and experienced before assignment. If the program is decentralized, the staff of the education department should be experienced, but a comparatively larger number of health educators located within the various units will need to be trained.

In a decentralized program, the director or coordinator of health education is responsible for selecting the health educators in the various units, but does so in close consultation with the director of each unit. Such selection should be based on personal visits with the staff members under consideration. An effective means of identifying staff members for consideration is to distribute a one-page questionnaire describing the program and requesting those interested to complete the bottom half of the form to be returned by a specific date. It is also useful to ascertain from discussions with a unit director who, if anyone, is already performing health education, has expressed an interest in it, has some training relevant to patient teaching, or has demonstrated the personality suitable for this educational role.

When staff members outside the education department have been selected to serve as health educators, their responsibilities need to be clarified. Salary adjustments, if any, need to be communicated, work responsibilities defined, and lines of reporting made clear. The staff members and two department heads involved need to be in agreement on these items at the beginning or problems may emerge. Such matters should normally be decided in writing to prevent later misunderstandings and possible grievances.

DEVELOPING A TRAINING PROGRAM

It is likely that the director or coordinator will have completed courses on staff development during his/her college training and will be familiar with the literature. The principles discussed in Chapter 3 regarding the development of health education programming can be modified slightly and used in planning a staff development program. However, a further review of major points is in order.

The beginning stage for planning a staff development program is to identify precisely the group to be trained. It is important to know, not only names, but also, training, work experience, and individual competencies. Such data can then be matched to job requirements in order to determine specific training needs.

Flexibility must be a part of staff development programs. Not all staff need to possess the same skills or competencies and not all staff learn at the same speed or in the same way.

A recommended strategy is to establish basic requirements for the position and provide an orientation to these responsibilities and skills. A variety of alternatives can then be made available to individuals wishing to increase their competencies, including guided self-study, attendance at conferences and workshops, completion of courses from nearby colleges or universities, team teaching or other situation-based practicums, and one-on-one counseling and instruction. As common needs are identified among the staff, inservice sessions can be established.

A personal development plan which will identify learning needs along with specific resources and activities to meet those needs, should be prepared by each staff member. The director or coordinator should stimulate and assist such planning, provide possible resources to meet these goals, and keep the plan on file. These plans can be the basis for the development of a comprehensive staff development program, while forming the foundation for developing a competent, dynamic health education staff.

CONCLUSION

Staff selection and training is critical to the development of a health education program that is both effective and efficient. Program planners would do well to remember that, "A chain is only as strong as its weakest link." It is important to remember that non-educational specialists will participate in health education programs. Physicians, nurses, therapists, technologists, technicians, and others all have important roles to play. Health education is a responsibility of all staff members and is not just within the purview of health education specialists. Yet, equally true, these specialists are needed on the team to plan, implement, and evaluate programs. They are also needed to deliver some of the services and to assist other members of the health care team to both recognize their opportunities to perform health education and develop the necessary techniques to offer patient instruction.

REFERENCES

Houle, Cyril. *Continuing Learning in the Professions*. San Francisco: Jossey Bass, 1980.

Tobin, Helen M.; Wise, Pat S. Y.; and Hull, Peggy K. *The Process of Staff Development*. St. Louis: C. V. Mosby Company, 1979.

Chapter 6

Determination of Needed Programs and Curriculum Development

6

INTRODUCTION

Attention has previously been directed toward establishing an appropriate structure within the hospital that will enable health education programs to develop most efficiently. After creation of policy statements and job descriptions, and training of staff, it is time to develop actual health education programs. A variety of considerations affect where to begin.

STRATEGIES

Several strategies may be used to help determine starting points. One way is to use existing programs and to refine procedures. For example, if a diabetes education program is currently in place but is poorly written up, conducted inconsistently, or is not approved by appropriate personnel, an important initial step is to upgrade the course, achieving the desired standard. Often, this simply involves formally rewriting the diabetes program using as a model a program currently conducted effectively on an informal basis.

A second strategy is to develop programs where there is a high level of interest, especially if that interest is evidenced by key staffers. If physicians or the director of the coronary care unit want an educational component added to the care of postcardiac patients, then this is probably an excellent program to initiate. Having interest and support can make developing programs easier than trying to develop ones that are not wanted. Furthermore, the working relationship that develops can often make the creation of future programs easier. While educational directors do not always have to develop requested programs, it is often sound planning procedure to assist staff in developing programs that they want early on, to foster support and enthusiasm for other programs.

Yet a third strategy is to perform a community or institutional needs assessment, involving a variety of people in prioritizing prospective programs. This strategy often encompasses the first two strategies since existing or desired programs will usually be near the top of the list of a formal needs assessment. However, a needs assessment can be a time-consuming project. It is a good idea to begin refining existing programs or initiating a program where there is a high level of interest while conducting a needs assessment.

A word of caution is in order: developing a program in a "quick and dirty" fashion is risky at best. The first programs developed and implemented are examined more critically than later ones. There is often a temptation to be task-oriented just to implement a program. Care should be exercised that the process is not compromised so much that either the program or the process is legitimately subject to criticism.

Community Needs Assessment

The first step is to tour the service area. A drive through the area by members of the committee can help identify needed educational programs. A "traveling committee meeting" is one way of gathering such impressions.

The committee also should discuss other sources of information. Planners and other hospital administrators can be most helpful in this regard. The local health department often has useful data on file including documentations of need and documentations of effect as part of grant applications for state and federally funded health programs. Statistical profiles of the service community may also be available from the administrator of the local health department. Again, having a representative from the local health department on the hospital health education committee encourages awareness of and ready access to such data.

Health Systems Agencies (HSAs) also have been created nationally, at the state level, and regionally within states. They may serve a single highly-populated county, but more often serve several counties within a large geographical region. These agencies are created to perform comprehensive health planning at the local or regional level and a majority of those involved in the planning process must be the actual consumers of health services, rather than the providers. Their statements of needs, goals, and implementation plans are readily available. Undoubtedly, HSA's annual plans are currently available in every hospital, and staff members have been designated to work closely with the agencies. These plans affect many other aspects of hospital services and can also be used effectively in health education planning.

The local chamber of commerce may have data available on health problems or existing programs, as may the local library or public schools. Available data should be assembled, reviewed, and filed for inclusion as appropriate.

There are also some state and national sources of data that can be interpreted for local implications. Decennial census data contain information by county describing the population a hospital serves. Specific census reports are available from the public libraries or by writing directly to the US Bureau of the Census.

Vital statistics are also routinely collected and distributed through state health departments. Statistics on birth, death, disease, marriage, and divorce are readily available. Information on communicable and chronic disease incidence, as well as statistics on leading causes of death and disability, are also collected and distributed. Each state health department will have a designated department or center collecting, interpreting, and disseminating such statistics. Yearly data usually will be available in local health departments, except for information on communicable diseases, which is collected weekly.

The National Center for Health Statistics is a valuable source of vital statistics on the nation as a whole. The Center also maintains a staff and budget to perform surveys on specific problems of current interest, interpreting data and disseminating reports.

A brief review of this data offers a view of the context in which institutional planning should occur. Careful review reveals prevalent health problems and provides a detailed description of the demographic variable of the population the hospital serves. Such a review is most useful if described briefly and discussed by the planning team during an initial meeting. It is important to be able to condense and synthesize large amounts of data, yet still to be able to discuss in detail if necessary ramifications for local planners.

Institutional Needs Assessment

In ascertaining hospital needs, a valuable ally is the medical records librarian. Most hospitals have computerized records and can call up needed data. Intake and discharge diagnosis data are helpful, along with information on the demographic variables of the clientele admitted. Readmission data and information on emergency room use can be useful in documenting the need for education programs. Demographic descriptions can be obtained from medical records for all diagnoses. A cooperative relationship must be established with the records librarian in order to have access to such information. In some hospitals, computers may not be programmed to elicit such information or the necessary software may not be available. But computerized record keeping systems can be made to provide data in any form planners desire.

Data that is more difficult to obtain include those diagnoses made in the offices of private physicians and in clinics. Though some such records may be computerized, more often than not physicians will only be able to provide estimates, for instance of the number of diabetics, congestive heart patients, or stroke patients, that they see. Nonetheless, such estimates can provide useful information. Moreover, health education programs are intended to be preventive in scope and emphasis. It is, therefore, incumbent upon planners to consider patients whose illness has not necessitated hospital admission.

A series of interviews with area physicians can provide useful planning data, as well as presenting an opportunity to communicate with them information on program development. If the number of local physicians is too large for a personal interview, a brief questionnaire could be mailed. Exhibit 6–1 is an example of a survey that could be used as an interview schedule or as a mailed questionnaire.

It is also often of use to health education planners to gather impressions directly from patients about their educational needs and interests, and their perceptions of whether or not such needs are currently being met. Again, a simple survey can be administered to gather such data, either as an interview schedule or as a mailed questionnaire (Exhibit 6–2).

Data obtained from the several sources described above needs to be synthesized and analyzed by the planners. A filing system should be developed to make such data readily available while gaps in the information system need to be noted for future efforts. Planning must proceed using the data available, but efforts to improve the data-base for future planning is an important consideration.

Simply having data available does not ensure that the necessary decisions will be made. People still make decisions after reviewing the criteria and data. For example, one criterion for deciding which programs to develop may include simple frequency, however, planners may choose to focus on an entity with fewer cases but with more serious consequences. Planners may also begin programming for a disease with fewer cases but more opportunity for an educational intervention to bear an impact or, as stated earlier, on a problem where there is a high level of demand. The data does not dictate the decision but should at least be reviewed and be part of the decision-making process.

After a thorough analysis of educational needs, interests, and resources, a priority list of programs should be developed and made public as the basis of overall curriculum design. Interested parties should know what programs will be developed first and the rationale for such decisions. It is

Exhibit 6–1 Private Medical Practitioner Survey

Name____________________

Date____________________

Dear Doctor:

The health education staff at Community Hospital is attempting to determine the need for health education programs. We have reviewed census, area planning, and hospital diagnosis data. We also need some general impressions about patients being treated in private practice. Please provide an estimate of the number of your patients that might find educational programs useful in the following areas:

_____ Diabetes	_____ Postnatal care
_____ Heart disease	_____ Mastectomy
_____ Pacemakers	_____ Ostomy
_____ Prenatal care	_____ Preoperative

_____ Others (Please Specify)

In which of the above areas do you see the greatest need for hospital-developed programs for both inpatients and community members? Please list below.

If you would be willing to assist in developing or reviewing such programs, please indicate below which ones:

Any other comments about hospital-based health education programs will be appreciated. Please feel free to comment either on this form or directly to the hospital health education staff.

Please return the completed questionnaire within the next seven days to: Education Department, Community Hospital, Anytown, State. Thank you.

also appropriate to publicize that information to the community at large, since community resources will be used. Also, as stated before, such a decision has publicity value. Community members desire health education programs and will be interested in knowing what programs are being de-

Exhibit 6–2 Patient Survey on Health Education

Dear Patient:

Community Hospital is in the process of determining the need for additional health education programs for patients and members of their families. Your perceptions will be part of this assessment. Please respond to the following questions as accurately as possible.

__ Yes	__ No	Have you been admitted before for this condition or one related to it?
__ Yes	__ No	Have you ever attended any classes or educational activities to learn about your condition? If so, what?
__ Yes	__ No	Do you feel you adequately understand the following items: __ Your condition __ Your medication __ Dietary restrictions __ Activity restrictions __ Prescribed exercises and/or equipment __ Community resources
__ Yes	__ No	Do you feel your questions were answered fully, honestly, and accurately while you were a patient?
__ Yes	__ No	Would you be interested in attending a series of classes to more thoroughly explain any of the above matters, if it were available after discharge?
__ Yes	__ No	Do you feel there is a need for a series of classes to cover the matters identified above to be available for patients while in the hospital?
__ Yes	__ No	Do you have any other comments about the need for health education you would like to share? If so, please comment in the space below or on the back of this form.

Thank you for your participation. Please return the completed questionnaire within the next seven days to: Education Department, Community Hospital, Anytown, State.

veloped, who will be served, intended curriculum, and the proposed instructional timetable.

PROGRAM DEVELOPMENT AND CURRICULUM DESIGN

Target Group

The target group for any educational program should always be identified at the beginning of planning stage and should be described in as much detail as possible. The following two examples illustrate this need to be group specific. First, consider the differences in educational needs and interests of recently diagnosed juvenile diabetics as opposed to elderly, advanced diabetics. Second, think of a weight reduction program for those slightly overweight as opposed to a program for the obese. In each instance, both population groups need education and may share some needs but there are many other concerns and interests specific to their prognosis, age, and entry-level experience that might well dictate separate programs. As a rule, the more homogeneous the group, the more likely educational needs can be met.

A description of the target group in other ways is also important. Planners need to possess estimates of numbers that will be served. Specific decisions have to be made regarding family involvement in the program, because this affects the numbers, appropriate time frames, and content.

Goals

Planners must specify at the outset what is being planned and desired outcomes. It is imperative to agree on what members of the target group are to have accomplished in completing a program to plan effectively.

This planning begins with the development of rather general goal statements for the program, describing the desired long-range outcome of a program. For example, the goal of a diabetic education program might be: patients will be able to adequately perform self-care and generally manage their condition.

Objectives

Objectives are narrower in scope and are usually short-term. They describe in as detailed form as possible specific tasks to be learned. For example, an objective of a diabetic program might be: patients will be able to accurately read urine tests for sugar content.

Both goals and objectives can be written in a variety of formats, but the most generally preferred are those viewed from the perspective of the learner rather than instructor. Such objectives are usually termed behavioral or performance objectives, to indicate that the emphasis is on the response of the learner. Instructional objectives imply that the emphasis is on the educator. Though there is considerable variance in the use of terms and overlap in meaning, instructors must specify what the learner should be able to perform as a result of instruction.

Objectives are important for a number of reasons. First, and of most importance, they provide the basis for planning learning activities, selecting methods and materials, and organizing content. Teaching and learning are more effective if both the instructor and student have a clear idea of what is to be learned. A second reason for stating objectives clearly involves program evaluation, which will be discussed in detail in Chapter 11. It is difficult to accurately measure success if learning objectives are vague or stated in ways that do not readily permit measurement. The planning stage should take into consideration ways that learners can successfully demonstrate that the objective has been met.

Objectives need to be as specific as possible and use words that communicate the intended messages. In as much as they are behavioral objectives, they should use action verbs. Vague terms like "appreciate," "understand," "know," or "comprehend" should be avoided, because of the difficulty in verifying whether they have been met. More precise terms should be used such as "identify," "list," "demonstrate," "recognize," "apply," and "describe."

Three Domains of Learning

Behavioral objectives should be written in each of the three domains of learning—cognitive, affective, and psychomotor. Instruction has traditionally focused on the cognitive, which concerns intellectual processes. If it is appropriate for a patient to list, describe, interpret, recall, or differentiate, then learning is in the cognitive domain. Cognitive learning refers to a client's ability to demonstrate knowledge, comprehension, application, analysis, synthesis, and evaluation.

The affective domain focuses on feelings, attitudes, and values. Behavioral objectives of affective learning focus on making clients more receptive to new feelings, attitudes, and values; encouraging them to respond to those affective stimuli; and helping them to incorporate the new perceptions into their system of values. The affective domain involves awareness, willingness, preference, and commitment.

The psychomotor or action domain embraces observable behaviors, including neuromuscular motor skills, dealing with trial, adaptation, performance, and the regular practice of an activity so that it leads to development of a habit.

The example of promotion of regular exercise provides an understanding of how all three domains are needed in effective programming. Behavioral objectives should be written referring to the cognitive domain, such as, "clients will be able to list three positive effects of exercise on the cardiorespiratory system." Objectives also need to be written in the affective domain, such as, "clients will accept the need for exercise to be a regular and routine part of their life style." Proper knowledge and attitudes are conducive to the practice of regular exercise. Yet, the ultimate test of the program is in the action domain—"clients will engage in an exercise program at least three times-a-week."

Course Content and Schedule

Approaches vary on how detailed the course content should be in a curriculum. Some planners suggest a brief and general overview of the major topics to be addressed, leaving the specifics to those who perform the actual teaching. Other planners prefer to develop a detailed protocol of what is to be taught, so that instructors in each program cover the same material. This facilitates physicians prescribing only specific parts of the program. In a similar manner, patient educators can conduct their individual assessment of the learning needs of each patient and review or teach only certain sections as appropriate. Detailing what is to be taught also aids record keeping. However, creation of a detailed curriculum is a time-consuming process and one so developed will have to be kept up-to-date. The most difficult problem involved with that kind of specificity is securing agreement on precisely what is to be taught. The time involved in reaching that agreement can be vast.

Outlining the major concepts to be taught and describing the needs to be addressed are important parts of curriculum design regardless of the amount of detail developed. An example of a curriculum for asthmatic children and their families is presented in Appendix 6-A.

It is also important to consider the most appropriate method to teach each concept and to search for the most appropriate teaching materials. These can be detailed by groups of concepts or by individual concepts. A detailed discussion of the selection of methods and materials appropriate to the learning domains will be the focus of Chapter 7.

Consideration should be given to the most appropriate scheduling of the options available, and the preferred schedule should be identified. If a program can best be conducted in three sessions of 90 minutes, it should be so described. If it can best be done in four 30-minute presentations with family members present, that too should be planned. The appropriate schedule and emphases should be provided for those who will teach the material. While the recommendations, for a variety of reasons, will not always be followed, planners should at least be certain that those who use the material being developed are aware of desired outcomes.

CONCLUSION

The term "program" is often used by health educators to refer both to a hospital's entire set of educational activities and to a specific set of learning experiences focusing on a disease, disorder, or health promotion topic. In previous chapters, the discussion has emphasized the institutional focus, while in this chapter, the focus has been on more narrowly defined learning activities concentrating on a specific topic.

The sequence in which programs are developed is an important decision. The criteria and processes used in making such judgments are often as important as the decision itself. It is always important to develop programs that are perceived to be needed by key groups. However, in as much as various groups will have differing perceptions of what is needed, it is also critical for planners to be able to justify their decisions.

All programs must be carefully planned and described in sufficient detail so that they will be acceptable to most groups involved and likely to achieve the desired results. The concepts presented in this chapter and the next, while time-consuming to implement thoroughly, are vital to success and should be carefully considered by planners.

REFERENCES

Espenshade, Jean E. *Staff Manual for Teaching Patients about Diabetes Mellitos*, Chicago: American Hospital Association, 1979.

Implementing Patient Education in the Hospital. Chicago: American Hospital Association, 1979. (Chapter 8.)

McCormick, Rose-Marie Duda, Gilson-Parkevich, Tamar. *Patient and Family Education: Tools, Techniques, and Theory*. New York: John Wiley and Sons, 1979. (Chapters 2-4.)

Narrow, Barbara W. *Patient Teaching In Nursing Practice: A Patient and Family-Centered Approach*. New York: John Wiley and Sons, 1979. (Chapters 11-13.)

Pritchett, Sue. *Patient, Family and Community Health Education: Design and Management of Hospital Based Programs*. Atlanta: Pritchett and Hull Associates, 1977. (Pages 20–44.)

Redman, Barbara Klug. *The Process of Patient Teaching in Nursing*. 4th rev. ed. St. Louis: C. V. Mosby Company, 1980. (Chapter 4.)

Squyres, Wendy D., ed. *Patient Education: An Inquiry into the State of the Art*. New York: Springer Publishing Co., 1980. (Chapter 4.)

Zander, Karen; Bower, Kathleen A.; Foster, Susan D.; Towson, Marilynn C.; Wermuth, Mara Ruments; and Waldum, Karyl M. *Practical Manual For Patient Teaching*. St. Louis: C. V. Mosby Company, 1978.

Appendix 6-A

Family Asthma Class

A TEACHER'S GUIDE

There will be four 90-minute sessions in a two-week period. These sessions will be held on alternate week nights (M-W-T-Th) from 7-8:30 p.m. A ten-minute break midway through each session is suggested.

The Family Asthma Program is suggested for a group of six children and their parents. Children should be at least 7 years old and of similar ages if possible. Any other interested household member is welcome to attend. A physician will refer families to the program.

A respiratory therapist and whatever aids felt to be necessary for the program will be the primary instructors. A physician will be available during the third session for questions and answers. Other professionals that may be involved with the program include the physical therapist and the occupational therapist.

Materials to be used during these sessions include *A Learner's Guide,** pamphlets on asthma, a learning game developed for asthmatic children, the film "A Breath of Fun," and a textbook from which reading assignments

---

*Not included as part of this appendix. All material in that handbook is incorporated in this Teacher's Guide. In addition, this guide includes explicit instructions to educators on implementation of the asthma program.

may be given. It is recommended that the respiratory therapist use the book *Breathe Easy* as a resource. This is also recommended reading for each family. It is suggested that the community or hospital library have at least six copies on hand to loan to the Family Asthma Program participants and that copies be available should the family decide to purchase one. The pamphlet, *What Everyone Should Know About Asthma,* is intended primarily for children with asthma and can be obtained from the American Lung Association.

The first session will deal with the definition of asthma and an orientation to the program. Topics will include who gets asthma, anatomy and physiology, diagnosis, and general activity and asthma. A pretest and a medical history questionnaire are to be filled out during or previous to this session.

Living with asthma will be the topic of the second session. Dietary habits, housekeeping, pets, school age problems, treatment, exercise, and an explanation of general breathing exercises will be covered. At the end of this session a quiz will be given to the participants on information presented in Sessions I and II.

The third session will deal with accepting asthma. Medications will be discussed. A physician should be available for a question and answer period. The children will be involved in the learning game, and the film "A Breath of Fun" will be shown.

The fourth and final session will emphasize putting it all together. It will include a review and evaluation and some type of social event. Helping agencies available in the area should be discussed.

The Family Asthma Program can be held at almost any type of facility. It is suggested that wherever the sessions are held, it should be possible to divide the adults and children into two groups during the third session. A divided room or two adjoining rooms would work out the best.

Session I Overview of Asthma

Behavioral Objectives

Each family will be able to demonstrate its knowledge of asthma with 75% accuracy on a quiz covering the following five areas:

1. definition of asthma
2. anatomy and physiology of an asthma episode
3. who gets asthma
4. diagnosing asthma
5. general exercise

Suggested Activities

- Use the pretest in *A Learner's Guide*
- Complete the Patient Medical History Form in *A Learner's Guide*
- Lecture, and ask for questions and answers on the topics identified in objectives
- Obtain a model of the lungs from the American Lung Association to use for demonstration
- Consider use of an opaque or overhead projector to demonstrate anatomy and physiology of asthma (Refer to the illustration in *A Learner's Guide.*)

Pretest

(To be administered at beginning of Session I)

1. Does asthma usually cause lung damage?
2. What is asthma? What are the effects of asthma on the body?
3. What is an asthma episode like?
4. What happens inside the body during an asthma episode? Describe as thoroughly as you can the effects on specific body parts.
5. In the United States, about how many million people have asthma? (Hint: There are about 220 million people living in the US today.)
6. If a child has asthma, will he/she have it for the rest of his/her life? Why?
7. Can asthma be inherited from parents?
8. How does a person know if he/she has asthma?
9. For children who have asthma, what is an important thing to remember about the amount of exercise that is suggested?
10. Why are some things called triggers for asthma? What are some of these triggers?
11. Is everyone who has asthma subject to the same triggers?
12. Can asthma be cured? What can be done to help a person who has asthma?
13. When someone says that a drug has "side effects," what does he/she mean?
14. What particular kind of exercise is encouraged for asthmatics?
15. How does a person's mental and emotional state affect asthma?
16. What is the difference between intrinsic and extrinsic asthma?
17. What is the position in the body of the diaphragm, especially in relation to the lungs?

Patient Medical History

Instructions: Both the parents and the patient should fill this questionnaire out together.
All information is about the patient.

Date:_______
Age:_______

How long ago were you diagnosed by a physician as an asthmatic?

____

What medications are you presently taking, at what times, and in what amounts?

____

____

List all equipment presently being used in your home for asthma treatment:

____

____

What kinds of activity causes you to have shortness of breath, weakness, fatigue in your legs, or other problems?

____

____

Do you ever wheeze (whistle in your chest) when you breathe hard?
Yes ( ) No ( )
Are you bothered by a chronic cough? Yes ( ) No ( )
Do you use oxygen? Yes ( ) No ( )
What is your current treatment program? (For example, steaming, breathing exercises, IPPB, etc.)

____

____

Definition of Asthma

Asthma is a disease of the respiratory system. It is an overreaction to any one or a combination of things, mainly allergy-producing substances (allergens), respiratory infections, or emotional stress. The chief symptom of asthma is difficult breathing with or without wheezing and coughing. This is caused by a narrowing of the bronchial tubes from bronchial muscle spasms.

Allergic asthma is most often seen in children. When it occurs in the spring or summer, the cause of the allergy and asthma attack is usually pollen or mold. When allergic asthma does not follow a seasonal pattern, it is usually caused by dust, animal dander, food, or drugs. Respiratory infections are responsible for the development of an asthmatic attack in about 40 percent of asthmatics. These attacks occur in the winter when the greatest number of respiratory infections develop.

Asthma "attacks" occur at varying intervals, and between attacks, asthmatics are usually completely free of respiratory symptoms. There is no cure for asthma. However, there are many ways to control and prevent asthmatic attacks so that asthmatics can lead comfortable lives with little interference in daily activities.

Session II Living with Asthma

Behavioral Objectives

A. Each family will be able to demonstrate its knowledge of asthma with 75% accuracy on a quiz covering the following three areas:

1. material covered in Session I
2. treatment plans for asthma, including medication use
3. dos and don'ts of asthma

B. Each family will be able to demonstrate currently used relaxation breathing techniques.

Suggested Activities

- Lecture/Discussion. Refer to material on "Medication" and "Dos and Don'ts" in *A Learner's Guide.*
- Use bulletin board, chalkboard, or table display to show "Dos and Don'ts" of asthma.
- Demonstrate and practice relaxation breathing in class.
- Instruct families to prepare questions to ask the physician at Session III.

Medications

There are three common types of medication for asthma patients. These are bronchial dilators, antibiotics, and mucous thinners.

An aerosol is defined as a suspension of liquid or solid particles in air or oxygen; the process of forming an aerosol is called nebulization. The purpose of aerosols in the treatment of asthma is to deposit bronchial dilators directly on the respiratory track where a high concentration can be achieved and exert its effect.

Some trade names of bronchial dilators by routes of administration are:

- oral—amesec, quadrinal, and choledyl
- intravenous—aminopuylline
- rectal suppositories—aminophylluire
- inhalation—isupril, bronkosol, micronephrine, vaponiphrine

The pharmacological effect of the bronchial dilator drugs is the relaxation of smooth muscle spasm and shrinkage of mucous membranes. Some side effects are:

- tachycardia, palpitations, etc; anxiety, nervousness, tremor, and headache
- building-up sensitivity to a particular drug by overdosing or too frequent use
- rebound effect; benefit lasts 5–10 minutes and then difficulty in breathing returns more intensely than before

Some equipment for administration of bronchial dilators for inhalation are: (1) Bird, (2) Bennett, (3) Monogram, (4) Handi-vent, (5) Maxi-myst, and (6) Hand bulb nebulizer DiVilluss 40. Procedure for using nebulizer:

1. Prepare glass nebulizer. Remove both corks.
2. Measure 5 drops of bronchodilator in nebulizer.
3. Measure 10 drops of sterile water into nebulizer containing broncho.
4. Check nebulizer to be sure it puts out adequate mist.
5. Position nebulizer at mouth with mouth wide open.
   DO NOT CLOSE LIPS AROUND NEBULIZER.
6. Exhale.
7. Inhale a deep abdominal breath squeezing the nebulizer bulb *once* at beginning of inspiration.
8. Hold breath momentarily at peak of inspiration.
9. Exhale through pursed lips.
10. Repeat 7, 8, and 9 for total of 8 breaths.

Preparation of Sterile Water:

1. Boil water and storage container for 20 minutes.
2. Use only 3 days then discard and boil fresh water.

3. Refrigerate between use.

Procedure for Cleaning Nebulizer:

1. Wash with detergent and water after every use. Do not store left over medication.
2. Rinse well.
3. Let dry and store in plastic bag.
4. Once-a-day soak in vinegar and water solution (1 quart water with ¼ cup vinegar) for ten minutes. This controls water bacteria.
5. Shake off excess solution.
6. Let dry and store in plastic bag.

To rid the lungs of excess mucus, the administration of humidity is used:

1. Steaming equipment
   a. Cold-room humidifier and ultrasonic nebulizer
   b. Hot baby bottle-warmer, vaporizer, and facial sauna
2. Procedure for use
   a. Do this after using bronchial dilator.
   b. Breathe steam in through mouth. Nose filters out the moisture.
   c. Steam for 10 minutes, repeat bronchial dilator, steam again for 10 minutes.
3. Cautions in using steam
   a. Use with caution—may trigger an attack.
   b. Do not let water stand in large containers. There is danger of bacterial growth.

Antibiotics are used to lessen the chance of infection. They may be administered by the physician when the chance of infection is great (during the winter months). Asthma patients should try to avoid persons with colds. Getting a flu shot might prevent some infection.

Dos & Don'ts

Do see your doctor if you have trouble breathing or if you have complications of bronchitis, emphysema, or sinusitis.
Do try to avoid people with colds or flu.
Do get enough sleep. Adequate rest is important.
Do check with your doctor before beginning any exercise program.
Do avoid stressful situations. Asthma attacks can occur from stress.
Don't tire yourself out by overworking or playing too hard.

Don't watch thriller movies or exciting television programs that could result in an attack.
Don't drink a lot of alcoholic beverages. The grains contained in the alcoholic beverage could be harmful to you.
Do avoid grass, ragweed, and pollens; also mold and dust.
Do avoid foods, such as, eggs, milk, and wheat products.
Do avoid tobacco smoke.
Do avoid irritants caused by industry.
Do avoid cold air.
Do avoid extreme temperatures and/or humidity.
Do stay in altitudes of 300–600 feet above sea level.
Do consult your doctor before moving to a different climate.
Do know how to recognize an asthma attack:

1. Shortness of breath and wheezing may occur.
2. You must sit up to breathe.
3. The tissue of the neck tightens as a result of the struggle for air.
4. The chest expands due to the overinflated lungs because air cannot be expelled.
5. A person having the attack may appear blue in the face and lips due to a lack of oxygen.

Do know that asthma occurs when the branches of the "lung-tree" become too narrow for air to pass. Air becomes trapped in the tiny air sacs of the lungs and cannot be expelled.

Relaxation Breathing

PURPOSE: To understand and demonstrate the process of relaxation breathing. This breathing pattern should result in relaxed neck, shoulder, and chest muscles that will in turn facilitate easier breathing.
NOTE: Following a deliberate teaching procedure for relaxation breathing is important. The first half-hour should be spent:

1. Tell class what you are going to do.
2. Give them step-by-step content of relaxation breathing.
3. Rationalize the logic and motivate.
4. Show them how to do it.
5. Let them do the various steps in their seats with you.

In the second half hour have the patients practice the procedure over and over under your observation to make certain they do it comfortably and correctly. You will need tables for them to practice breathing while in the reclining position, long open space to practice while walking, and stairs for practice while climbing steps.

Ideal Breathing Pattern

1. Normally, breathing is automatic, uncomplicated, and unconscious. To teach control of breathing, we want the simplest, most effective pattern.
2. The pattern must be functional and one the patient will use with or without activity.
3. The pattern of breathing will keep the patient calm and relaxed in the event of breathing difficulties.

Relaxation Breathing Procedure

1. Overview of steps
   a. use abdomen to move air
   b. breathe out through pursed lips
   c. use prolonged exhalation
2. Abdominal pattern
   a. On exhalation, the stomach is drawn in. This pushes the diaphragm up.
   b. On inhalation, the stomach protrudes. This allows the diaphragm to move down. Air is drawn deeper into the lungs. The stomach action helps to increase the movement of the diaphragm and thus the movement of air. Continual movement of air will keep the patient relaxed.
3. Pursed lips on exhalation
   (Remember: breathe in through the nose)
   Results in slowing of breathing and thus relaxing the shoulder, neck, and chest muscles.
   Technique:
   a. Tighten lips as to blow out a candle.
   b. Should feel stream of air on hand six to eight inches from mouth.
   c. The roof in the back of mouth should arch slightly if done correctly.
4. Prolonged expiration
   Results
   a. Allows time to move air from the lung.
   b. Improves air exchange on each normal breath.
   Technique
   a. Establish breathing rhythm. Time for expiration should be at least twice as long as for inhalation.

   b. Most natural way is to allow two slow counts on inhalation and four counts on exhalation with pursed lips.
   c. Rhythm should be adjusted to each individual according to what is the most natural for him/her.
5. Positions for abdominal breathing pattern.
   Pattern is done in all positions, such as, lying, sitting, standing, walking, and climbing stairs.
   a. When walking, rhythm is adjusted with steps. Breathe in on two steps and breathe out on the next four steps.
   b. Procedure for climbing stairs is the same as for walking. This may need to be adjusted for those who climb stairs more slowly.
6. How to make breathing pattern automatic
   a. Practice pattern for 2–5 minutes, then breathe as usual. Repeat this procedure every hour.
   b. Practice in any position in which you find yourself.
   c. Acquiring the abdominal breathing is learning a neuromuscular skill. It takes time to train the muscles to function in a new way.
   d. Don't become discouraged. It will take six weeks to four months of continual practice before it becomes automatic.

Posttest

(To be administered at the end of Session II)

1. Does asthma usually cause lung damage?
2. What is asthma? What are the effects of asthma on the body?
3. What is an asthma episode like?
4. What happens inside the body during an asthma episode? Describe as thoroughly as you can the effects on specific body parts.
5. In the United States, about how many million people have asthma? (Hint: There are about 220 million people living in the US today.)
6. If a child has asthma, will he/she have it for the rest of his/her life? Why?
7. Can asthma be inherited from parents?
8. How does a person know if he/she has asthma?
9. For children who have asthma, what is an important thing to remember about the amount of exercise that is suggested?
10. Why are some things called triggers for asthma? What are some of these triggers?
11. Is everyone who has asthma subject to the same triggers?
12. Can asthma be cured? What can be done to help a person who has asthma?
13. When someone says that a drug has "side effects," what does he/she mean?

14. What particular kind of exercise is encouraged for asthmatics?
15. How does a person's mental and emotional state affect asthma?
16. What is the difference between intrinsic and extrinsic asthma?
17. What is the position in the body of the diaphragm, especially in relation to the lungs?

Session III Emotional Acceptance

Behavioral Objectives

A. The parent will be able to recognize the importance of emotional acceptance and define the part it plays in the overall treatment of the disease process by participating in a discussion with a panel of experts, including:

- physician (must be at least one present)
- therapists
- counselor
- minister
- pharmacist

B. The child will be able to recall facts related to him/her through the film, *A Breath of Fun.*

C. The child will be able to participate in a learning game which emphasizes the "Dos and Don'ts" of living with asthma.

Suggested Activities

The children will be taken to a separate area and shown the film and then will play the learning game. A discussion followed by a question and answer period should occur immediately after the film and the game.

The adults will participate in a panel discussion with resource person(s). Any questions can be directed to physicians at this session.

The instructor may wish to use problem solving or role playing techniques as a way of demonstrating problems associated with the emotional acceptance of asthma.

The film, *A Breath of Fun,* is recommended for use in Session III. It is available from the Asthma and Allergy Foundation of America, 801 Second Ave., New York, New York 10017 (212)867-8875. Films are not available for purchase. Rental fees should be submitted with the request, several weeks in advance. *A Breath of Fun* is a 16mm color, sound, 18-minute long film that depicts the experience of asthmatic children during a program of exercise and respiratory rehabilitation. The management and treatment of the asthmatic child must be comprehensive, and the whole child must be treated in his or her natural environment. With this in mind, the film shows how a course of exercise and games, as a physical fitness program, can be an important auxiliary to medical treatment.

Other audio-visual material available from the Asthma and Allergy Foundation of America include: *Nothing to Sneeze At,* a 16mm, color, sound, 13½-minute long cartoon, which highlights the scope of the allergy problem; its nature, causes, and varieties of symptoms and treatments. The film is designed to reach a wide lay audience ($10). *What You Should Know About Asthma,* is a 40-slide show with a 10-minute cassette tape which describes asthma and other allergic diseases outlining methods of control and treatment. For adult lay and professional audiences ($5).

Feel free to use audio-visual materials from other sources you may locate.

Session IV Putting It All Together

Behavioral Objectives

A. The parent will be able to participate in a discussion with the instructor outlining the available helping agencies and resources (educational and financial) as they relate to the asthma patient.

B. The child will be able to recall facts related to him/her through the film *A Breath of Fun,* and/or the learning game, and/or the crossword puzzle.

C. Each family will be able to demonstrate correct procedures associated with maintaining their home care breathing equipment.

D. Each family will be able to participate in a discussion with the instructor about any questions or concerns they may have from Sessions I, II, ad III.

Suggested Activities

- Review first, presenting highlights of the last three sessions, then opening up to class discussions and questions.
- Discuss various helping agencies in the area. Give names, services, and telephone numbers.
- Demonstrate correct procedures for maintenance of breathing equipment.

- Use Course Evaluation.
- The instructor may want to plan a social hour at this last meeting.

Glossary

abscess—collection of pus surrounded by tissue.
aerosol—a fine mist that can be inhaled. Medicines are often given as an aerosol.
allergen—a substance that induces an allergic reaction.
allergy—a sensitivity to some normally harmless substance.
alveoli—small air sacs at the end of bronchial tubes where gas exchange takes place.
anaphylactic—rapid, exaggerated allergic response.
antibiotic—substance produced by a microorganism or manufactured through chemicals to slow, stop the growth, or kill a disease germ.
antibody—substance already present in the body to fight infection.
antigen—protein or carbohydrate substance that stimulates the production of an antibody.
bacteria—organism that can produce infection.
belly breathing—breathing with the use of abdominal muscles and diaphragm along with chest muscles.
bronchial dilator—medicine to help open up the bronchial tubes when they are congested or tight.
bronchitis—inflammation of bronchial tubes.
bronchogram—chest x-ray film made after filling bronchial tube with radio opaque material.
bronchospasm—constriction of air passages by spasmodic contraction of bronchial muscles.
bronchospirometry—measurement of vital capacity of each lung by an instrument called a spirometer.
capillaries—smallest blood vessels located in the walls of the alveoli, they bring blood that takes oxygen from the air in the alveoli and gives up carbon dioxide.
carbohydrates—one of six essential nutrients (e.g., sugar).
carbon dioxide—a waste gas in used air that is removed from the body in breathing out.
chronic—long-lasting, repeated, continuous (said of illness).
cilia—hair-like extensions with wave-like motion located in an air passageway moving mucus out of the lungs and into the windpipe and esophagus. Cigarette smoking can definitely harm the cilia and interfere with mucus removal.

constriction—act of drawing together; tightening.
cyanosis—blueness of skin due to a lack of oxygen.
diaphragm—a dome-shaped muscle forming a floor to the chest cavity and separating it from the abdominal cavity.
diaphragmatic training—exercises to help the patient make better use of the diaphragm in breathing.
dilation—spreading apart; opening.
elimination diet—diet restricted to a few normally nonallergenic foods, followed by testing of individual foods, one at a time.
emphysema—disease of lungs causing loss of elasticity; getting rid of the used air and breathing in fresh air is difficult.
esophagus—swallowing tube through which food travels from mouth to stomach.
exhale—to breathe out.
extrinsic asthma—asthma caused from outside agents, such as, weather and inhalants.
gas exhange—the giving-up of carbon dioxide and the picking-up of oxygen by the blood as it passes through the lungs.
generic—a group of medicines available for common use, not protected by trademark.
genetics—science of heredity.
hay fever—allergic nasal reaction sometimes accompanied by asthma.
hereditary—transferred from parent to child by genes.
infection—an invasion by germs, viruses, or other organisms.
inflammation—the swelling and other changes in tissue caused by an infection, irritation, or injury.
inhalation therapy—treatment prescribed by a doctor in which medicine in the form of gas (such as oxygen or liquid droplets is breathed into the lungs).
inhale—breathe in.
intravenous injection—medication administered by a needle into the veins.
intrinsic asthma—asthma having causes other than allergies. (Example—respiratory or other infections).
IPPB—Intermittent Positive Pressure Breathing; breathing with the help of a machine to take fresh air in and to keep the tubes open for breathing out.
lobes—sections of the lungs. The right lung is divided into three lobes, the left into two.
metabolism—the chemical changes in living cells by which energy is provided for body functions.
mixed asthma—where causes are extrinsic and intrinsic.

mucus—clear, slippery fluid produced by the tissue lining the bronchial tubes.
nebulizer—an appliance that creates a fine spray of fluid (such as medicine) so that it can reach deep into the lungs when breathing in.
negative skin test—where injection of a substance under the skin does not result in a raised bump, and the person is not allergic to that substance.
oxygen—a colorless, odorless, and tasteless gas in air; necessary for life.
perennial—infection of lung tissue.
postural drainage—helping to clear mucus out of the bronchial tubes by the position of the body; by having the head lower than the lungs.
predisposition—condition of being inclined, having a tendency.
pulmonary function tests—tests to find out how well the lungs are working.
pus—yellow-white matter produced by an infection, consisting of fluid, broken-up tissues, blood cells, and germs.
rales—wheezing or other sounds when air passes through a narrowed passage or one containing moisture.
residual air—"stale air" not expelled after a deep breath.
respiration—the process of breathing; inhale and exhale.
respiratory tract—the breathing system, including the nose, throat, windpipe, bronchial tubes, and alveoli.
side effects—undesirable condition from the use of the drug.
spasm—a sudden constriction or tightening.
sputum—phlegm; the fluid matter brought up with coughing and then spit out, may consist of mucus, pus, or both.
sputum culture—test to determine contents of sputum.
suppository—medicine in a bullet-shape made of wax-like material, to be placed in the rectum, where the material melts and is absorbed.
symptom—evidence of disease or physical disturbance.
timed vital capacity—amount of air expelled in one second.
trachea—windpipe; the largest air tube, leading from mouth to lungs.
triggers—physical or chemical conditions or substances that initiate an asthma attack.
ventilation—the process of getting air in and out of lungs.
vital capacity—amount of air brought into the lungs and expelled in one respiration.

Family Asthma Self-Care Class Program Evaluation

Asthma Overview (Session I)

1. Was the material in this session on what asthma is and how it affects your lungs new information for you? yes ( ) no ( )

2. If no, where did you get your information?
   Physician ( ) Therapist ( ) Reading ( )
   Other ( ) explain ________________________________
3. If yes, was the information presented in such a manner that you could explain asthma and how it affects the lungs to someone else? yes ( ) no ( )
4. Have the general exercises been of any help in cutting down or lessening possible episodes? yes ( ) no ( )

Living With Asthma (Session II)

1. Did the list of dos and don'ts provide you new areas of familiarity thus lessening the chance for an episode? yes ( ) no ( )
2. Has the instruction on relaxation breathing been helpful in your normal daily routine? yes ( ) no ( )
3. Did the quiz covering Sessions I and II help you to focus in on the major points of these sessions? yes ( ) no ( )
4. Was the quiz a fair measure of what should have been learned up to that point? yes ( ) no ( )

Emotional Acceptance (Session III)

1. Do you understand what type of medication your child uses and why? yes ( ) no ( )
2. Was the question and answer period with the expert panel of value to you? yes ( ) no ( )
3. Did the experts satisfactorily answer your questions? yes ( ) no ( )
4. Did the learning game provide new information on living with asthma? yes ( ) no ( )

Putting It All Together (Session IV)

1. Could any of the helping agencies or resources be contacted for assistance to your family? yes ( ) no ( )
2. Have these sessions given you a better understanding of your asthma? yes ( ) no ( )
3. What session was the most valuable to you? ________________

   Why? ____
4. Was the material presented in such a way that the whole family could benefit?

Crossword Puzzle with Key

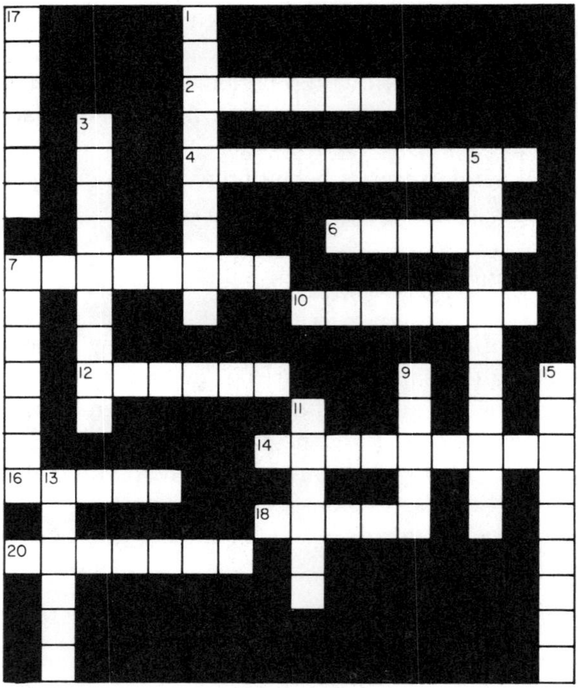

Down

1. muscle that separates the chest cavity from the abdominal cavity
3. appliance that creates a fine spray of fluid (such as medicine)
5. the process of breathing; inhale, exhale
7. a fine mist that can be inhaled
9. clear, slippery fluid produced by the tissue lining and bronchial tubes
11. to breathe in
13. colorless, odorless, and tasteless gas in air; necessary for life
15. act of drawing together; tightening
17. fluid matter brought up with coughing and spit out

Across

2. disease of respiratory system
4. transferred from parent to child by genes
6. a factor in causing an "attack"
7. substance that induces an allergic reaction
10. long-lasting, repeated, continuous
12. to breathe out
14. an invasion by germs, viruses, and other organisms
16. sections of the lungs; the right lung is divided into three, the left into two
18. wheezing or other sounds caused when air passes through a narrowed passage or one containing moisture
20. evidence of disease or physical disturbance

(*Answers are on page 95.*)

Session I yes ( ) no ( )
Session II yes ( ) no ( )
Session III yes ( ) no ( )
Session IV yes ( ) no ( )

5. Would you like more sessions or a follow-up? yes ( ) no ( ) If yes, covering what? ______________________________
____
6. Would you recommend these classes to others with asthma? yes ( ) no ( )
7. Do you have any comments or suggestions about the classes? _____
____
____

THANK YOU!

Key

Down	*Across*
1. diaphragm	2. asthma
3. nebulizer	4. hereditary
5. respiration	6. stress
7. aerosol	7. allergen
9. mucus	10. chronic
11. inhale	12. exhale
13. oxygen	14. infection
15. constriction	16. lobes
17. sputum	18. rales
	20. symptom

Chapter 7

Selection and Use of Educational Methods and Materials

7

INTRODUCTION

There is a tendency for people to "teach the way they were taught rather than the way they were taught to teach." That is unfortunate since most people's teaching experience occurred in either the public schools or in colleges and universities with young people. Teaching adults can and should be different as will be explored in detail in Chapter 12. Also, teaching in a hospital setting can and should be different from teaching in a high school or college. The methods that are used are one important way that this teaching may differ. Consideration of how to select teaching methods will be the focus of this chapter.

PROVIDING AN EDUCATIONAL MIX

Just as there is a natural tendency to teach as taught, there is also a tendency to develop a teaching method that works well for the teacher and then to stick with it. Unfortunately, for a variety of reasons, one teaching approach is rarely always effective. Plans should be developed for several educational strategies so that the learning needs of both individuals and groups are more likely to be met.

Variety is important for interest as well as effect. If attention is held by a different approach, concepts can be reinforced. As a general rule, the more of the senses that are used in the learning process, the more probable that learning will occur and will be retained. Accordingly, it is important for clients to hear the health educator explain why a problem might develop if the directions are not followed precisely. The client should visually see that same concept explained in charts and diagrams. While it might be inappropriate to have patients actually experience a problem as a teaching tool, there are ways of simulating such perception or of having the problem experienced vicariously through the media. Again, stated in generalities, the more actively involved in the learning process the learner is and the greater the mix of educational methods that is employed, the more learning is enhanced.

Educators, therefore, need to select a variety of methods and be comfortable with each. Likewise, educators should strive to present the same material using more than one method. Concepts presented in a lecture should be reinforced by a film, while material covered in a group discussion session should be reinforced with a pamphlet or flier. Educators should also be comfortable in selecting from a variety of methods as new situations dictate. Time, convenience, and the educational needs and preferred learning methods of clients can all be used as factors in choice of a method. Certainly learning is more likely to be enhanced if the methods are appropriate to the needs and interests of the target group, appropriate to the given situation, and varied.

RELATIONSHIP TO LEARNING OBJECTIVES

Methods should be carefully chosen according to the objectives of the lesson. As discussed in the previous chapter, learning objectives can be in the cognitive, affective, and psychomotor domains. If indeed, the objective is to teach content, then methods should be selected that are best at getting across knowledge. Lectures, pamphlets, films, or individualized teaching sessions can all be effective. Teaching aids can also help reinforce facts.

If the objective is to teach in the affective domain and impact on values and attitudes, methods again need to be chosen accordingly. Learning in these cases should be active, and other people should often be involved. Attitudes are "caught easier than taught." Discussions, counseling sessions, or other interactions with people with positive attitudes can be planned. Films, videotapes, and other teaching aids can also be used to allow some of this to be captured vicariously.

If, for example, the objective is to teach a mastectomy patient to have a positive image of herself, then interaction with former mastectomy patients who have made the adjustment should occur in person or by film. The role model effect can have considerable positive impact on an anxious patient. The interaction with someone who has experienced a mastectomy, and who will not only understand but will respond openly and honestly to questions, will have more impact on attitudes than simply having a staff member talk to the patient about her concerns. Again, the choice of a teaching method used should be affected by the learning objective.

There is also considerable advantage in getting several patients together and getting them talking to each other. Such "support groups" can be of enormous value when patients are at different stages of development. Problems that one patient is facing may have already been coped with by others who will offer helpful suggestions. Likewise, a question that one patient asks may be something that another patient would not think to ask until a later time when a staff member isn't present. But perhaps the most important value of such support groups is the effect they have on other patient's attitudes. When patients realize that they are not alone and that others have coped with their condition, then levels of hope increase, spirits rise, and prognosis improves.

If the learning objective is in the psychomotor domain, the teaching is usually best done one-on-one. The needed skill should be demonstrated after which the patient should be supervised in trying it. Individual attention is usually more efficient and more effective in skill development than group demonstrations. For example, if the objective is to teach a chronic lung patient how to use a piece of equipment that is to become part of his/her inhalation therapy, then that discussion could best be done on an individual basis.

RELATIONSHIP TO TARGET GROUP

The educational needs and preferences of clients should be a major factor in choosing which methods to use. The age group, socio-economic level, prior schooling, and prior educational activities with the disease should all be factors.

If for example, a 70-year-old patient is readmitted for complications and had already been through the material, then a short film or a bedside visit might serve as adequate review. If the patient is forty and a registered nurse, again only a review or a response to questions might be necessary to focus in more detail on identified problem areas. If on the other hand, the patient is newly diagnosed, then the full range of educational activities might be in order depending on the patient's existing knowledge. Again, if the patient is a juvenile, the methods used might be quite different than if the patient is a senior citizen.

Regardless of age, reading ability is also an important variable. Functional illiteracy is still a problem in most counties in this country. Reading ability is severely limited in some patients, irrespective of their age.

Methods used will also vary in convenience and ease of use. Preparation and required "lead time" will vary. Some methods are more time-consuming than others. Classes have to be scheduled for outpatients around the varying schedules of several individuals. Some methods are too time-consuming or inconvenient for the clients to enjoy. For example, a busy staff member might be willing to read a book, but not be willing to attend classes.

Also of significance is the fact that clients have preferred methods of learning. Even though a client is able to read, it may be the least preferable means of learning. Such a client might prefer to see a film. Some might be turned off to classes as they remember them in school, while others may remember school favorably and enjoy attending a series of classes. Some clients might enjoy the attention of an individual visit with a health educator, while others might prefer the anonymity of a group. Others might enjoy the socialization that is part of a group experience and be willing to learn and share in this manner. When preferred methods of learning are used, learning increases.

METHODOLOGIES

It is, therefore, important to the extent possible to give learners a choice of learning methodologies that are consistent with the learning objectives. The more commonly used methods and a brief description of them include:

- *Audio-visual* methods appeal to the senses of hearing and sight and support other instructional methods employed by the teacher.
- *Creative projects* allow learners to engage in constructive and creative learning activities. A variety of the senses are involved, and learning occurs through the practical application of knowledge.
- *Demonstrations* enable the learner to observe and experience a concept in a tangible, concrete form.
- *Discussion* involves various forms of verbal interaction between the teacher and the learners or among the learners themselves. Usually, the teacher will provide general directions to discussion activities.
- *Brainstorming and problem solving* encourage the learners to think for themselves and apply solutions to a number of problems.
- *Role playing and dramatization* enhance understanding and interest through simulated learning situations.
- *Games* serve the dual purpose of gaining learner interest while relaying health information. Games are better used as a supplement to other educational information and techniques.
- *Field trips* allow learners to observe actual examples of information presented in the class.

- *Resource speakers* usually increase the practicality and relevance of classroom instruction. However, it is important that the teacher be certain that the guest speaker will make an acceptable presentation.

- *Lectures* generally enable teachers to present what they consider to be important information in a short period of time without distraction or interruption. The drawbacks of lectures, however, are that they limit the learner's personal involvement and creative thinking.

Modules or learning packages can be developed for individual or group use. They can be repeated, used with supplementary material, or used individually for a quick review. The methodologies ultimately used should represent a combination of the best educational choice and the learner's preference.

EFFECTIVE USE OF AUDIO-VISUAL AIDS

There is a natural tendency for educators to rely heavily on films, tapes, cassettes, etc. Certainly, they can be an effective teaching tool when used appropriately. A later section in this chapter will include a more detailed discussion of the factors involved in selecting such teaching aids. However, a chapter on methods would not be complete without at least a brief discussion of the abuses of media as a teaching method.

A film or a videocassette is a teaching aid, not an educational program. It is an aid to an educator, not a substitute for teaching. There are institutions where grant money has been used to purchase videocassette units and a series of videocassettes have been obtained. The program as planned is for every patient to see the cassette, either on a monitor wheeled to the bedside, or on the room's closed-circuit television set. Such programs are often ineffective for a variety of reasons. The staff member bringing in the cassette unit may leave the room. If the patient is in a ward, a television might be on; company may be present, talking and laughing; and staff members may be coming and going causing frequent interruptions. The fact that a program has been shown to a client does not mean that any learning has occurred.

This is also a problem for staff development educators. They videotape a lecture to be viewed by staff on the second and third shifts who could not attend the original presentation. Often all that is required is to sign the sheet stating that they have viewed the program, even though their minds and sometimes their bodies may be involved in other matters.

Audio-visual methods can be effective if encompassed in a well-developed program rather than made to substitute for such a program. Educators must guard against over simplistic approaches.

When media is used as part of a program, there are several other considerations that come into play. The film, tape, or whatever should be previewed and carefully selected to be appropriate for the intended group. Appropriateness should include consideration of the content, level, and general relevance of the material. Material might be appropriate in content and level, but focus on urban settings rather than rural areas, or Caucasian populations rather than ethnic ones. It is more difficult for the relevance of content to be established when the setting is irrelevant to the participants.

When a good audio-visual aid is chosen, it needs to be adequately introduced. Viewers need to be instructed what to look for, what they will be seeing, and what is important. Of most importance is the follow-up discussion. Clients should be encouraged to ask questions, which should be addressed as openly as possible. Key questions should also be posed by the educator to ascertain if the viewers learned the major concepts. Questions can also be posed in a way to stimulate discussion, or to see if the clients will be able to apply the materials to future home life settings.

Audio-visual aids are not intended to stand alone, even though they are often misused in that manner. They should be carefully selected, adequately introduced, and followed-up with discussion of the major points to be learned. When used in that matter, they can be a most effective teaching method.

SELECTION AND USE OF EDUCATIONAL MATERIALS

There are no simple guidelines that will describe which material to use in a given educational setting or for a given client. There is, however, a continuing need for variety and flexibility. No single item will be of interest to all learners, nor will it have lasting impact. There is an ever-growing abundance of patient education material on the market, available from both commercial and public service organizations. A variety of methods and materials that promote active learning and involve several of the senses is necessary for effective long-lasting learning to occur. Likewise, the best combination of educational methods and media for one learner or group of learners is not necessarily the best combination of methods for others.

Sources of Educational Materials

An important starting place in the selection of educational materials is to determine what is available and to file this information for ready access when needed. Most sources of educational material have publication lists or catalogs and are happy to send free copies. Most also have mailing lists that enable educators to stay current. Indeed, hospitals are often on such mailing lists whether they want to be or not.

There are four general sources of material that may be useful: (1) voluntary health agencies, (2) government agencies, (3) pharmaceutical companies, and (4) commercial educational companies. First, and often most valuable is the voluntary health agencies, like the American Cancer Society, the American Heart Association, etc. All such organizations have national offices, most have state or regional offices, and some have local offices, especially in urban areas. Initial contact can be made at any level and is usually most appropriate at the local or state office. Inquiries made at the national office will be referred to state or local affiliates for processing when possible. Appendix 7–A provides a selected list of voluntary health agencies with complete addresses. Educational material from these agencies is usually available free or at low cost. Large quantities may require reimbursement for printing costs, unless there is an agreement to cosponsor a program.

A second important source of educational materials is government agencies. Of major interest are federal clearinghouses. Clearinghouses collect, describe, and catalog educational material in a variety of ways. They issue newsletters or other fliers on available materials to those on their mailing list. Usually such materials will be on specific areas of interest. They also respond to requests of all kinds, either by phone or mail. The agencies are generally well-staffed, and the material is on line in data banks, so that requests can be handled promptly. Appendix 7–B lists several clearinghouses according to area of interest.

State and local health departments are also excellent sources of educational materials. State health departments usually have a staff of production people who develop high quality material to meet specific current needs. Film libraries are often available at the state level as well.

Local health departments are usually a repository of materials from other sources that are used in local programs to meet specific area needs. Occasionally, materials are produced locally. Most importantly, city or county health departments usually have educational material available locally to meet local needs. Sharing relationships can often be worked out, especially if health department staff are involved in the hospital's health education program in other ways.

A third important source of materials is the various pharmaceutical companies and other commercial firms that supply hospitals. It is often necessary to work with the purchasing office to make contact with these people, because they often do not get through the hospital. A simple request to purchasing that the education department be notified when a sales representative is in the office can be of enormous benefit in building a library of materials.

It is also appropriate to contact such firms directly. Firms that supply medication or supplies for the disease being programmed for will usually have educational materials on that disease. An inquiry simply addressed to that company and the attention of the education department will usually get it to the right people and result in them contacting you directly. Materials available from such companies are usually free, though some advertising will inevitably be present. Appendix 7–C presents a selected list of pharmaceutical companies that may be useful to contact.

Yet a fourth source of educational materials is commercial organizations (Appendix 7–D) who sell educational materials for the profit involved. While the material may often be expensive, some excellent and innovative materials have been made available that should not be overlooked. Such organizations are especially good for more expensive materials like films, video tapes, models, etc. They also have free catalogs and mailing lists.

Selecting the Right Teaching Aid

When looking through the myriad of material for the right teaching aid, the major consideration should always be the group of clients for whom it is intended. As discussed in earlier chapters, it is important to describe present or potential clients as accurately as possible. At minimal, a client's age, sex, ethnic background, and socio-economic status should be factors in selection of appropriate teaching aids. The second and equally important factor in selecting the aid is the behavioral objective for the learning activity. Indeed, only when a group of prospective learners have been identified, and it is known rather specifically what is to be taught to that group, can a good final decision be made on educational material.

There are a multitude of other considerations that enter into the decision as to what is the best teaching aid. Exhibits 7–1, 7–2, and 7–3 call several such considerations to mind.

While on the subject of audio-visual aids, the topic of equipment should be addressed. Purchase of audio-visual equipment is a serious matter that should only be made after considerable thought has been given to it by a variety of people. The following items are among those that deserve attention:

- *Cost*: Continuous design programs may require larger expenditures.
- *Adaptability*: The program design should be flexible enough that multi-programs can use the same equipment.

Exhibit 7-1 Worksheet Evaluating Printed Materials

Title ______________________ Author ____________

Publisher ______________________________

Cost __________ Date of publication ______________

Language written in ______________________

Purpose or theme ________________________

For what groups is this material appropriate? (Check all appropriate.)

Men ____ Women ____ Pediatric ____ Geriatric ____

Cultural groups ______________________

Occupational groups ______________________

A B C D Audience appeal: Does it get attention, lead the reader on, keep attention?

A B C D Accuracy: Is it accurate and up-to-date?

A B C D Approach: does it agree with the emphasis and approach used locally?

A B C D Organization: It it logical, clearly developed, easy to follow, believable?

A B C D Completeness: Sufficient detail; too much detail?

A B C D Tone: Personal, supportive, positive, honest?

A B C D Physical properties: Is layout, print, illustrations, and color appropriate for the intended group?
Is it attractive?

A B C D Graphics: Simple, clear, enough?

A B C D Vocabulary: Is vocabulary familiar or explained for readers?

A B C D Readability: Short sentences, clear plain language, jargon avoided.

Grade Level ____________

(Grade level can be easily checked by using the Gunning Fog Index. In any 100-word sample, count the number of sentences, and compute the average number of words per sentence. Count the number of words with three or more syllables, and add that number to the average number of words per sentence. Multiply that number by 0.4. The product translates directly into a grade level.)

Strengths:

Weaknesses:

Recommendation:

Signed: ______________________ Date: ______________

- *Serviceability*: The technical equipment may need spare parts (bulbs, fuses, etc.) that will be required as back-up equipment.

- *Purchase vs. lease*: Larger pieces of equipment may have a short life due to innovative improvements in the field, therefore, leasing would guarantee improvements are kept timely. Service repair contracts usually accompany lease agreements. Only purchased items can be depreciated.

- *Degree of training*: If the equipment considered requires specialty technicians, then probably it's too expensive a venture. If the training of the patient on how to use the teaching machines is too complicated that it overshadows the patient education program material, then the most elaborate of equipment would be wasteful.

- *Objectivity vs. promotion*: Equipment and teaching materials should remain objective and informative in content, not laced with brand-name sales and promotions.

- *Hidden extras*: Does the package price include all the pieces that are necessary for a starting program, or are there software pieces that are called "optional" or extras that really are mandated for larger pieces in order to be fully utilized.

- *Audience appeal*: Considering the target group and their skills and acceptability is very important when selecting brochure materials, videotape, and similar group teaching methods.

- *Back-up or alternate programs*: Time is a very important commodity for the patient as well as the professional. If there is a power failure or machine breakdown, an alternate script or equipment must be available. (Can the machine work on a battery source as well as house current.)

- *Durability*: The machine or material must withstand the passage of time and the stress of various patient handlings.

- *Manufacturer availability*: Even the best of equipment needs care and repair, therefore, the distance of manufacturer to classroom may be prohibitive for optimal service with minimal time delays.

- *Documentation*: Is the machine fully or conditionally warranted and guaranteed? Are there other similar machines in operation at neighboring institutions that can be polled for advice and consent?

- *Trial periods*: Sales demonstrations are not similar to classroom utilization, therefore, a 90-day trial program may be warranted.
- *Inhouse storing areas*: Once equipment is accumulated, is there an organized tagging and storing system for these pieces of equipment? Do you have a "loan-out" policy established?
- *Trade-in value/updated materials*: Is there a market for you to unload your antiquated equipment for cash or apply to purchase price of newer equipment? Does the printer of your brochure and programming material have periodic up-date sessions to enable timeliness in the presentations?
- *Program scheduling*: Can the class be appropriately scheduled between neighboring institutions so that suitable equipment and speakers can be utilized on a sharing basis?

Using Teaching Aids Effectively

Educational materials are intended to be teaching aids and should accordingly be used as part of the educational program, not in lieu of a program. It is easy to give "lip service" to health education by handing out pamphlets.

Health educators have on occasion been labeled as "pamphlet pushers" because of the emphasis given to educational material. Other health educators have reacted in the opposite direction and rarely use materials. As is so often the case when the pendulum swings, the prudent course of action is between these two extremes.

Effective health education should include the use of a variety of teaching aids that should be used in a variety of ways. They can be used to introduce a topic so as to give the overview, before focusing attention on some of the specific parts. They can be used to teach the basics and to focus attention and interest, so that students and instructor are all considering the same concept. Charts and diagrams are especially good to use as handouts, i.e., take home material to focus attention, emphasize sequence, and provide the basis for later review.

Educational material can and often should be used to review or reinforce material discussed in previous sessions. Instructions and their rationale should be given in writing to each client so as to maximize learning and review.

The use of overhead projectors and other audio-visual equipment can also provide flexibility and variety and increase the effectiveness of edu-

Exhibit 7-2 Worksheet Evaluating Posters and Charts

Title ______________________________

Publisher ______________________________

Cost __________ Approximate size __________ Language ______

Purpose or theme ______________________________

For what group is this material most appropriate. (Check all that apply.)

Men ____ Women ____ Pediatric ____ Geriatric ____

Specific cultural groups ____________________

Specific occupational groups ________________

A B C D Appeal: Does it get attention quickly; hold attention?

A B C D Physical properties: Artwork, lettering, color, etc.

A B C D Accuracy: Accurate and contemporary?

A B C D Balance: Not symmetrical, but size and color is compensated for.

A B C D Movement: Center of interest not centered; flows in sequence.

A B C D Unity: Close together or tied together so as to appear a whole.

A B C D Simplicity: Only necessary elements; small elements grouped so as to reduce their apparent number.

A B C D Clarity: Good lettering, enough contrast; understood at a glance.

A B C D Color intensity: Attention-getting colors are yellow, orange, red, green, blue, indigo, violet. Colors read most easily at a distance are dark blue on white, black on yellow, white on red, black on yellow, green on white, blue on white.

A B C D Color appropriateness: Red, orange, and yellow attract and excite; green, blue, and purple are soothing, cool, and restful; light colors appear to increase the size of objects while dark colors appear to decrease size. Blue, green, and red are the most generally preferred colors.

Strengths:

Weaknesses:

Recommendation:

Signed: ____________________

Date: ____________________

Exhibit 7-3 Worksheet Evaluating Audio-Visual Aids

Title ______________________________

Subject ______________________ Date ____________

Publisher ______________________________

Purchase Price ______________ Rental ______________

Type of Media

- __ 16mm film
- __ 35mm slides
- __ 8mm film loop
- __ videotape __ reel __ cassette
- __ audiotape __ reel __ cassette
- __ slide tape program
- __ transparencies
- __ other
- __ Color __ Sound __ Time

Purpose or theme ______________________________

For what group is this material most appropriate. (Check all that apply.)

_____ Men _____ Women _____ Pediatric _____ Geriatric

Specific cultural groups ______________

Specific occupational groups ______________

A B C D Appeal: Does it get and hold attention?
A B C D Physical properties: Photography and sound?
A B C D Accuracy: Accurate, up-to-date?
A B C D Approach: Does it agree with approach used locally?
A B C D Organization: Logical easy to follow?
A B C D Completeness: Sufficient detail; too much detail?

Strengths:

Weaknesses:

Recommendation:

Signed: ______________________

Date: ______________________

cational materials used. Courses or books in audio-visual aids can provide insight into such use. Sales representatives from commercial distributors are also very willing to provide consultation in such matters.

CONCLUSION

Educational materials can enhance a health education program a great deal, if they are properly used. Appropriate selection and use can make a program appear professional or amateurish. They can add considerably to the cost of a program or can be quite inexpensive. They can enhance learning and retention or can actually inhibit it, if improperly selected or used.

Decisions made regarding educational materials ought not to be made by one person and ought not to be taken lightly by the staff. While materials might not necessarily make or break a program, they are in fact a tremendously important component that can add interest and create enthusiasm. When there is interest and enthusiasm in learning the necessary content that has been carefully organized and planned, significant learning always occurs.

REFERENCES

Lazes, Peter M., ed. *The Handbook of Health Education.* Rockville, Md.: Aspen Systems Corporation, 1979. (Chapters 8 and 10.)

McCormick, Rose-Marie Duda, and Gilson-Parkevich, Tamar. *Patient and Family Education: Tools, Techniques, and Theory.* New York: John Wiley and Sons, 1979. (Chapter 2.)

Narrow, Barbara W. *Patient Teaching In Nursing Practice: A Patient and Family-Centered Approach.* New York: John Wiley and Sons, 1979. (Chapters 14 and 15.)

Redman, Barbara Klug. *The Process of Patient Teaching in Nursing.* 4th rev. ed. St. Louis: C. V. Mosby Company, 1980. (Chapters 6–8.)

Squyres, Wendy D., ed. *Patient Education: An Inquiry into the State of the Art.* New York: Springer Publishing Co., 1980. (Chapter 5.)

Appendix 7–A

A Selected List of Voluntary Health Agencies

Allergy Foundation of America, 801 Second Avenue, New York, NY 10017
American Academy of Family Physicians, 1740 West 92th Street, Kansas City, MO 64114
American Academy of Pediatrics, 801 Hinman Avenue, Evanston, IL 60204
American Cancer Society, 777 Third Avenue, New York, NY 10017
American Dental Association, 211 East Chicago Avenue, Chicago, IL 60611
American Diabetes Association, One West 48th Street, New York, NY 10020
American Diabetic Association, 430 North Michigan Avenue, Chicago, IL 60611
American Foundation for the Blind, 15 West 16th Street, New York, NY 10010
American Group Practice, PO Box 949, Alexandria, VA 22313
American Heart Association, 7320 Greenville Avenue, Dallas, TX 75231
American Hospital Association, 840 North Lakeshore Drive, Chicago, IL 60611
American Lung Association, 1740 Broadway, New York, NY 10019
American Medical Association, 535 North Dearborn Street, Chicago, IL 60610
Arthritis Foundation, Inc., 475 Riverside Drive, New York, NY 10027

Epilepsy Foundation, 1828 L Street NW, Washington, DC 20036
Metropolitan Life Insurance Co., Health and Welfare Division, One Madison Avenue, New York, NY 10010
Muscular Dystrophy Association of America, 810 Seventh Avenue, New York, NY 10019
National Association for Mental Health, 1800 North Kent Street, Arlington, VA 22209
National Council on Aging, 1828 L Street, NW, Washington, DC 20036
National Easter Seal Society for Crippled Children and Adults, 2023 Ogden Avenue, Chicago, IL 60612
National Foundation March of Dimes, Box 2000, White Plains, NY 10602
National Multiple Sclerosis Society, 257 Park Avenue South, New York, NY 10010
National Society for Prevention of Blindness, 79 Madison Avenue, New York, NY 10016
Parkinson Disease Foundation, 640 West 168th Street, New York, NY 10032
Pharmaceutical Manufacturers Association, 1155 15th Street, NW, Washington, DC 20005
Planned Parenthood, 810 Seventh Avenue, New York, NY 10019
United Cerebral Palsy Association, 66 East 34th Street, New York, NY 10016
United Ostomy Association, 1111 Wilshire Boulevard, Los Angeles, CA 90017

Appendix 7–B

Selected Federal Health Information Clearinghouses and Information Centers

AGING
National Clearinghouse on Aging
202/245-2158
330 Independence Avenue, SW
Washington, DC 20201

ALCOHOL
National Clearinghouse for Alcohol Information (NCALI)
301/468-2600
PO Box 2345
Rockville, MD 20852

ARTHRITIS
Arthritis Information Clearinghouse
301/881-9411
PO Box 34427
Bethesda, MD 20034

Source: National Health Information Clearinghouse, prepared under contract issued by The Office of Health Information, Health Promotion, Physical Fitness, and Sports Medicine, Washington, D.C., September 1980.

CANCER
Cancer Information Clearinghouse
National Cancer Institute
Office of Cancer Communications
9000 Rockville Pike, Building 31, Room 10A18
Bethesda, MD 20205

Office of Cancer Communications (OCC)
301/496-5583
Public Inquiries Section
9000 Rockville Pike, Building 31, Room 10A18
Bethesda, MD 20205

CHILD ABUSE
Clearinghouse on Child Abuse and Neglect Information
202/755-0590
PO Box 1182
Washington, DC 20013

CONSUMER INFORMATION
Consumer Information Center
303/323-9301
Pueblo, CO 81009

DIABETES
National Diabetes Information Clearinghouse
202/842-7630
805 15th Street, NW, Suite 500
Washington, DC 20005

DIGESTIVE DISEASES
National Digestive Diseases Education and Information Clearinghouse
703/522-0870
1555 Wilson Boulevard, Suite 600
Rosslyn, VA 22209

DOMESTIC VIOLENCE
National Clearinghouse on Domestic Violence
301/428-3104
PO Box 2309
Rockville, MD 20852

DRUG ABUSE
National Clearinghouse for Drug Abuse Information
301/433-6500
PO Box 416
Kensington, MD 20795

EMERGENCY MEDICAL
National Clearinghouse for Emergency Medical Services
301/436-6267
PO Box 911
Rockville, MD 20852

FAMILY PLANNING
National Clearinghouse for Family Planning Information
301/881-9400
PO Box 2225
Rockville, MD 20852

FOOD/DRUG
Food and Drug Administration (FDA)
301/443-3170
Office for Consumer Communications
5600 Fishers Lane, Room 15B–32 (HFE–88)
Rockville, MD 20857

FOOD NUTRITION
Food and Nutrition Information Center (FNIC)
301/344-3719
National Agricultural Library Building, Room 304
Beltsville, MD 20705

GENETIC DISEASES
National Clearinghouse for Human Genetic Diseases
301/279-4642
1776 East Jefferson Street
Rockville, MD 20852

HANDICAPPED
Clearinghouse on the Handicapped
202/472-3796
330 C Street, SW
Washington, DC 20202

HEALTH EDUCATION
Bureau of Health Education (BHE)
404/329-3235
1300 Clifton Road, Building 14
Atlanta, GA 30333

HEALTH INDEXES
Clearinghouse on Health Indexes
301/436-7035
National Center for Health Statistics
Division of Analysis
3700 East-West Highway
Hyattsville, MD 20782

HEALTH INFORMATION
National Health Information Clearinghouse (NHIC)
703/522-2590 in VA
800/336-4797
PO Box 1133
Washington, DC 20013

HEALTH PLANNING
National Health Planning Information Center (NHPIC)
301/436-6736
3700 East-West Highway, Room 6–50
Hyattsville, MD 20782

HEALTH STANDARDS
National Health Standards and Quality Information Clearinghouse (NHSQIC)
301/881-9400
6110 Executive Boulevard, Suite 250
Rockville, MD 20852

HIGH BLOOD PRESSURE
High Blood Pressure Information Center
301/652-7700
120/80 National Institutes of Health
Bethesda, MD 20205

INJURIES
National Injury Information Clearinghouse

301/492-6424
5401 Westbard Avenue, Room 625
Washington, DC 20207

MENTAL HEALTH
National Clearinghouse for Mental Health Information
301/443-4513
Public Inquiries Section
5600 Fishers Lane, Room 11A–21
Rockville, MD 20857

OCCUPATIONAL SAFETY
Clearinghouse for Occupational Safety and Health Information
513/684-8326
4676 Columbia Parkway
Cincinnati, OH 45226

PHYSICAL FITNESS
President's Council on Physical Fitness and Sports
202/755-7478
Washington, DC 20201

POISON CONTROL
Division of Poison Control, FDA
301/443-6260
5600 Fishers Lane
Rockville, MD 20857

PRODUCT SAFETY
Consumer Product Safety Commission
800/638-8326
800/492-8363 in MD
800/638-8333 in AK, HI, VI, PR
Washington, DC 20207

RAPE INFORMATION
National Rape Information Clearinghouse (NRIC)
301/443-1910
5600 Fishers Lane, Room 11A–22
Rockville, MD 20857

REHABILITATION INFORMATION

National Rehabilitation Information Center (NARIC)
202/635-5822
4407 Eighth Street, NE
Washington, DC 20017

SMOKING
Office on Smoking and Health
301/443-1575
Technical Information Center
5600 Fishers Lane, Room 116
Rockville, MD 20857

SUDDEN INFANT DEATH SYNDROME (SIDS)
Clearinghouse for Sudden Infant Death Syndrome Information and Educational Material
703/522-0870
1555 Wilson Boulevard, Suite 600
Rosslyn, VA 22209

SURGICAL OPINION
National Second Surgical Opinion Program
330 Independence Avenue, SW
202/245-1845
800/638-6833
800/492-6603 in MD
Washington, DC 20201

Appendix 7-C

A Selected List of Major Pharmaceutical Manufacturers with Patient Education Programs and Materials

Abbott Laboratories Hospital Products Division Dept. 976 AP6B Abbott Park North Chicago, IL 60864	Total Parenteral Nutrition I.V. Infusion Products Catheters and Tubing
Alcon Laboratories, Inc. 6201 South Freeway Box 1959 Ft. Worth, TX 76101	Ophthalmic Preparations Contact Lenses Glaucoma Cataracts
Ames Company Division Miles Laboratories, Inc. 1127 Myrtle Street Elkhart, IN 46514	Urine Testings Diabetes
Arnar-Stone Laboratories 601 East Kensington Road Mount Prospect, IL 60056	Perianal Care Hypotension

ATCO Surgical Supports 450 Portage Trail Cuyahoga Falls, OH 44222	Prosthesis Braces
Ayerst Laboratories Division of American Home Products 685 Third Avenue New York, NY 10017	Tension Anxiety
Bard Consumer Products C.R. Bard, Inc. 741 Central Avenue Murray Hill, NJ 07974	Colostomy Ileostomy
Barnee-Hind Ophthalmic Products 895 Kifer Road Sunnyvale, CA 94086	Glaucoma Cataracts Contacts
Burroughs Wellcome Co. 3030 Cornwallis Road Research Triangle Park, NC 27709	Tolerance/Pain
Chesebrough-Ponds, Inc. Hospital 33 Benedict Place Greenwich, CT 06830	Hygiene
Ciba Pharmaceutical Co. Div. Ciba-Geigy Corp. 556 Morris Avenue Summit, NJ 07901	Tension/Anxiety Arthritis
Davol Inc. Box D Providence, RI 02901	Colostomy Products Prosthesis
Dentur-Eze Co. Division of Blistex, Inc. 700 Enterprise Drive Oak Brook, IL 60521	Oral Hygiene

DeVilbiss Medical Products Division Somerset, PA 15501	Inhalants Humidifier Care
Dista Products Co. Division of Eli Lilly & Co. Box 1407 Indianapolis, IN 46206	Diabetes
Drustar Unit Dose Systems, Inc. 1385 Brookham Drive Grove City, OH 43123	Health Care Facilities Medication Compliance
Eaton Laboratories Division Norwich Pharmaceutical Co. 17 Eaton Avenue Norwich, NY 13815	Nutrition
Endo Labs, Inc. 1000 Stewart Avenue Garden City, NY 11530	Anticoagulant Therapy
Hoechst-Roussel Pharmaceutical, Inc. Route 202-206 North Somerville, NJ 08876	Hypertension
Hollister-Stier Labs 3525 North Regal Street Box 3145 Term. Annex Spokane, WA 99220	Allergies
Johnson & Johnson, Health Care 500 George Street New Brunswick, NJ 08901	Child Care First-Aid
Parke Davis & Co. Joseph Campau Avenue At the River Detroit, MI 48232	Angina Control
Upjohn Company 7171 Portage Road Kalamazoo, MI 49002	Diabetes

Appendix 7-D

A Selected List of Commercial Sources of Patient Education—Hardware and Software

Channing L. Bete Co., Inc.
45 Federal Street
Greenfield, MA 01301 (413) 774-2301

American Learning Systems, Medfact
Division of American Family Cancer Plan, Inc.
PO Box 2173-31902
1106 Jeanette Avenue
Columbus, GA 31906 (404) 327-2619

American Learning Systems
Nurse Aide Training
John L. Venet
27911 Ursuline
St. Clair Shores, MI 48081

Audio-Visual Products
Lansford Publishing Company
1088 Lincoln Avenue

PO Box 8711
San Jose, CA 95155 (408) 287-3105

Career Aids, Inc.
5024 Lankershim Boulevard, Dept. 7F
North Hollywood, CA 91601 (213) 985-5656/985-5659

Cassettes Unlimited
(Health and Patient Services)
Roanoke, TX 76262 (817) 430-1084

Cinema Medics
664 North Michigan Avenue
Chicago, IL 60611 (312) 664-6170

Teach 'em Inc.
Dept. C-5
625 North Michigan Avenue
Chicago, IL 60611 (312) 787-0303

MEDEX
444 Northeast Ravenna Boulevard
Seattle, WA 98115 (206) 543-6483

Media Library Programs
Clinton Memorial Hospital
Education Department
805 South Oakland Street
St. Johns, MI 48879

Rexton Medical Visuals (RMV)
1007 Andrus
Lansing, MI 48917 (517) 321-2023

Research Media, Inc.
4 Midland Avenue
Hicksville, NY 11801 (516) 433-5672

Research Media, Inc.
96 Mount Auburn Street
Cambridge, MA 02138 (617) 661-9150

OMNI Education
190 West Main Street
Somerville, NJ 08876 (201) 524-1501

Professional Research, Inc.
660 South Bonnie Brae Street
Los Angeles, CA 90057 (800) 421-0200

Milner Fenwick, Inc.
3800 Liberty Heights Avenue
Baltimore, MD 21215 (310) 664-2600

Physicians Art Service, Inc.
343-B Serramonte Plaza Office Center
Daly City, CA 94015 (515) 994-1150

Pavis
Box 566
Leeds, AL 35094 (800) 633-8632

National Educational Media, Inc.
15760 Ventura Boulevard TWX/Telex: 910–495-2033
Encino, CA 91436 (213) 990-2125

SPENCO Health Education Catalog
SPENCO Medical Corporation
PO Box 8113
Waco, TX 76710 (800) 433-2400

Pelican Films
3010 Santa Monica Boulevard
Santa Monica, CA 90404

Chapter 8

Self-Help Programming

8

INTRODUCTION

There is seldom enough time for staff to meet all the health education needs of patients and their families, other employees, and members of the community. Fortunately, it is not necessary or appropriate to do so. Most adults are self-directing and would prefer to learn on their own. Indeed, many health improvement activities are done because of individual rather than staff initiative.

Yet it is possible for staff to maximize utilization of self-help groups. At least two approaches are possible: (1) self-help programs can be incorporated into hospital health education programs or (2) direct referrals can be made to community programs. Both approaches are important to effective utilization of self-help strategies that are the focus of this chapter.

DEFINITIONS

Several terms are commonly used, the most common of which are self-care, patient activation, and self-help. Self-care is the most narrowly defined term and is interpreted literally. *Self-care* refers to programs that teach clients to care for themselves whenever and wherever they need health care. It traditionally includes first aid training and preparation for returning home from a health care institution. More recently, the concept has been enlarged to include self-initiated and applied preventive efforts.

Self-care proponents currently stress self-monitoring; self-treatment whenever possible; self-sufficiency; and, in general, self-control. Advocates attempt to elevate the needs and interests of the person above the needs and interests of health care professionals and institutions. They prefer to emphasize the needs perceived by patients themselves and would deemphasize compliance with physicians' orders. They attempt to avoid "blaming the victim" for behaviorally induced problems, and instead stress the decision-making role of the individual by endeavoring to maximize choices. The self-care movement has grown very rapidly and has a large number of proponents.

Patient activation is somewhat different in focus but includes much of self-care. It refers specifically to an educational program initiated in Georgetown University which trains patients and prospective patients to take a more active role in their health care. Traditionally, health care providers such as doctors and nurses have been active, and consumers have been passive recipients of their care. An activated patient is one who is trained to monitor symptoms, use self-care activities whenever possible, and seek the services of specialists when necessary. An activated patient continues to play a partnership role during medical treatment for that condition.

Self-help encompasses both self-care and patient activation and refers to the consumer who performs activities formerly reserved for providers. More specifically, self-help refers to a lay person who is trained to function on his or her own behalf or lay people organized to help each other. This most inclusive term is used in this chapter, though all are appropriate.

RATIONALE

Inasmuch as self-help programming is not usually a major part of hospital health education, a rationale will be presented. While this rationale is important for all to understand, it is recognized that for many only a brief review will be necessary.

It should be noted that the concept of self-help programming is not a new one, even though the terminology may have come into common use only in recent years. Since the beginning of time people throughout the world have cared for their own health needs as best they could and have been quick to care for others who were ill.

Treatment for disease has become more complex and often requires medical specialists. While the origins of medicine go back several thousands of years, the biggest advances have been made in the last century. As the practice of medicine increased in complexity, the role of the specialized health care provider expanded, and the role of the consumer decreased. The advocates of self-help believe that it is time for the pendulum to swing back to a larger role for the consumer. Stated more formally, the movement to elevate the role of self-help comes as part of efforts to take the mystery out of medical care, to return care to the consumer, and to take much of it back to the home setting from which it came.

Self-help proponents do not presuppose that traditional medical treatment and concurrent hospitalization are safe. Self-care proponents call attention to "iatrogenic illnesses," such as, the side effects of treatment or problems that result from the direct effects of mistreatment. Proponents also refer to "nosocomial infections" that are picked up from the environment during hospitalization. Both can often be avoided through self-care.

Another major factor that contributed to the emphasis of self-care has been the shift in the causes of morbidity and mortality from the more acute communicable diseases to the chronic degenerative diseases. Physicians can cure a bacterial infection rather quickly, regardless of what the patient does, by appropriate use of antibiotics. Treatment of chronic disease, on the other hand, is usually a long-term process, and patient cooperation is usually integral to effective treatment. Even more importantly, many chronic diseases like diabetes do not have a cure per se, and the goal of treatment is to establish an acceptable maintenance plan with which the patient can live. The shifting emphasis from "curing" to "caring" has contributed to the increased attention to self-help programs.

The medical system also has other limitations. Self-help programs have demonstrated their ability to be more effective than traditional modalities for some disorders, as in the case of Alcoholics Anonymous. There is credibility in self-help programs where consumers have experienced the disorder which the patient is currently experiencing. The rehabilitation of an alcoholic or a mastectomy patient can be enhanced if the credibility and modeling effect of a successfully recovered patient are involved.

The concern about runaway health care costs is also part of the rationale for expanding self-help programming. The health care system has been described as underfinanced, understaffed, and underemployed. Many consumers are without adequate insurance coverage and are unable to purchase the needed health care. Likewise, many rural areas are designated by Health Systems Agencies in their comprehensive health plan as "medically underserved areas." People living in such areas may be as much as an hour's drive from primary medical care. Access to health care is often not convenient in time or place. Self-care is especially important in such isolated areas.

Yet another aspect of this issue is the underutilization of the health care system because of nonfinancial reasons. A general lack of confidence in treatment, personnel, programs, and facilities exists in many people's minds. The strong "self-help ethic" is a viable alternative for health care needs to some people.

There is yet another dimension to the rationale for self-help programming that surfaces when people are organized to help others: the benefit that accrues to the "helper." As one source has noted:

> (1) The helper is less dependent; (2) the helper in attempting to change or help the helpee becomes involved in persuading himself or herself while in the process of convincing the other; (3) in struggling with the problem of another person who has a like problem, the helper has a chance to observe his/her problem at a distance; (4) the helper obtains a feeling of social usefulness by playing the helping role.[1]

AVAILABLE PROGRAMS

Self-help programs come in a variety of forms with literally dozens of groups being available. No attempt will be made to be comprehensive in listing them in this chapter. Instead, a brief effort will be made to categorize such programs and to list examples of programs available in each category.

Primary care groups. There are groups formed whose mission is to provide the first contact with the treatment system. The group may or may not offer treatment modalities, as in the case of Alcoholics Anonymous or the various substance-abuse encounter groups. They may also be concerned with prevention and casefinding, such as the American Cancer Society's program on "Breast Self-Examination." Other examples include Emphysema Anonymous, the Arthritis Foundation, and the American Diabetes Association.

Support groups. Patients with chronic diseases often need the support of others who are fighting or have fought the problems associated with their disorder. Health education staff can easily organize support groups to meet these needs, which are often more emotional than physical and can best be met in social settings. Examples include Mended Hearts, Stroke Club, United Ostomy Association, and Reach to Recovery.

Behavior Modification Groups. The third type of self-help programs are those primarily concerned with behavior modification. Examples include Smokenders, Weight Watchers, TOPS, adult fitness programs, and stress reduction programs.

Certainly there are many other programs, and there are also organizations that don't fit readily into the above categories. Such a description can and should, however, stimulate thinking regarding self-help programs that are needed and available locally.

EMERGING STAFF ROLES

If the nature and effectiveness of self-help programs centers on the "people to people" aspect of them, what then should the role of health education staff be? In the literature, a basic concern is expressed that the program not be coopted by staff, thus lessening its effectiveness. The volunteer nature of it should be allowed to continue uninterrupted. However, when any volunteer programs are incorporated into a hospital's programs, staff roles emerge.

Health education staff need to be alert to the need for self-help programs and solicit groups to provide the necessary services. Administrative approval is usually needed, and staff can facilitate this process.

Existing groups may not be available locally, and an appropriate staff role may be to help recovered patients get organized and trained to provide the services. Likewise, programs may be available in other parts of the country, and a local chapter simply needs to be established.

Another important staff role is to educate other members of the staff about the new program. Professionally trained staff will typically have many questions and concerns about a volunteer program, which should be handled before the program is initiated. Another basic staff role is that of general supervision. There may be problems that develop, if, as an example, former deviants are used in a hospital.

Staff can and should anticipate problems and prevent or alleviate them. Volunteers need to be trained and supervised regarding the distinction between medical roles and volunteer roles. Provision for orientation activities is an important role, as is the screening of prospective volunteers. Not everyone should be allowed access to patients or employee groups. Volunteers should be sufficiently recovered and adjusted for a long enough period of time so as to be good role models. They should also have enough emotional stability to assist with the distraught clients that they may encounter.

Volunteers should be assisted in the administrative duties of their jobs. Teaching materials should be available, facilities reserved, and refreshments provided. Records should be kept and the role of the volunteer should be facilitated as much as possible. If there are unnecessary problems that additional staff support could have circumvented, volunteers are apt to discontinue participation in the program.

Another important staff role is to give appropriate recognition to volunteers. This may take the form of publicity, which is beneficial to both the institution and the volunteer, certificates, recognition lunches, etc. Volunteers need to feel appreciated, feel that they are making a useful contribution, and feel they are being supported by staff. If these three elements are in place, literally thousands of hours of volunteer labor can be built into a hospital's program.

The use of volunteers in a hospital-based program is not without problems. The biggest problem centers on locus of responsibility. If an outside group is brought into a hospital to conduct a program, is the group responsible for its own activities or is the hospital? If there is disagreement on content or procedures, can changes be forced by the hospital?

It goes without saying that programs should be thoroughly reviewed before being incorporated, so that problems can be anticipated and if possible avoided. Likewise, arrangements should be put in writing, perhaps in contract form; reviewed by general counsel; and signed by legal representatives. In the absence of such a contract, hospital staff should be present and in charge at all times, with it clearly understood that the outside groups are there as guests only, conducting their programs under the supervision of the staff. Contracts become imperative if commercial groups, such as, Weight Watchers or Smokenders, are brough in to use hospital facilities for a program directed specifically to hospital patients, staff, or the community.

If health educators opt to simply refer patients to outside groups, the referral needs to be in writing so as to increase the probability of follow-through. The referral form should include at least the name and address of the organization and the name and phone number of a person to contact. Other information like meeting time, cost, etc. are helpful. Attaching a promotional brochure to the referral form also enhances the likelihood of follow-through.

CONCLUSION

The role of the professional involved in self-help programs is similar to roles in other health education programs. Staff should plan, implement, and evaluate good self-help programs and facilitate the work of the volunteers. Though there may be problems, the risks are minimal compared with the results. Self-help programs can extend the capabilities of staff, and most importantly, be more effective in helping patients. They can and should be an important part of any hospital health education program.

NOTE

1. Alan Gartner and Frank Riessman, "Self-Help Models and Consumer Intensive Health Practice," *American Journal of Public Health,* August 1976, pp. 783–786.

REFERENCES

Gartner, Alan, and Riessman, Frank. *Self-help in the Human Services.* San Francisco: Jossey Bass, 1977.

Lazes, Peter M., ed. *The Handbook of Health Education.* Rockville, Md.: Aspen Systems Corporation, 1979. (Chapters 10–13.)

Levin, L.S.; Katz, A.H.; and Holst, E. *Self Care, Lay Initiatives in Health.* New York: Prodist, 1976.

Squyres, Wendy D., ed. *Patient Education: An Inquiry into the State of the Art.* New York: Springer Publishing Co., 1980. (Chapters 11–13.)

Vickery, Donald, and Fries, James. *Take Care of Yourself: A Consumer's Guide to Medical Care.* Reading, Pa.: Addison Wesley Publishing Co., 1978.

Chapter 9

The Hospital's Role in Community Health Programming

9

INTRODUCTION

For too long, hospitals have functioned independently of other community health agencies, serving as islands of health care in the midst of a community. Such isolation is disappearing. Hospitals have an opportunity, and according to the AHA, an obligation to play a leadership role in such programming.[1] The AHA has established a division which focuses on health promotion activities within the community, entitled "The Center for Health Promotion." It publishes a newsletter called *PROmoting HEALTH*,[2] which provides assistance to hospitals moving into such efforts. An overview of community health education opportunities that have been successful is the focus of this chapter.

DISCHARGE PLANNING

A traditional role of hospitals in the community setting has been and continues to be in the arena of discharge planning. It is considered a part of comprehensive health care by the Joint Commission on Hospital Accreditation. As the term suggests, it focuses on preparing the patient to either return to the home environment or be transferred to another health care facility. It is literally the preparation of the patient for discharge from the hospital.

Discharge planning usually has an educational component, though it is not limited to the education process. It usually involves a staff member with a background in social work who works with selected patients who need special arrangements to successfully leave the hospital. Examples of patients needing discharge planning include: (1) amputees, (2) quadraplegic and paraplegic patients, (3) older patients with chronic conditions, such as, stroke, heart attack, and emphysema, (4) any patient with a complicated treatment therapy that must be continued on a maintenance basis, and (5) patients who come from an inadequate home environment. Patients must be screened and referred by the doctors or nurses, or the discharge planner must routinely review the files of patients to be discharged to ascertain which ones need such help.

Education of patients and their families can alleviate some potential problems. Topics of discussions may include insurance or other financial considerations; activity restrictions; recommended diet; medications; purpose, use, and maintenance of in-home equipment; and obtaining medical supplies. Discharge planning should usually include written instructions for all of the above. If necessary, specific appointments for return visits to the outpatient department, to the personal physician's office, or to appropriate community agencies should be made. Referral to patient education classes is appropriate and should also include specific appointments.

It is obvious that discharge planning will often have to involve those family or friends caring for the patient and should very often be done, at least in part, in a joint session with the patient and family member. The planning should be informal, in the sense that there is adequate rapport and time for the patient and family to discuss whatever is of concern to them. It is likewise of importance to maintain written records and to provide follow-up as staffing permits. A telephone call in a few days to determine if all is going well is usually time well-spent. Including a telephone number for patients or their families to call when difficulties arise is also important, but needs to be planned for when staffing is available.

Referral to home health care programs in some hospitals or health departments is often appropriate, or to the Visiting Nurses' Association if available. Referral to a variety of commercial organizations that have provided satisfactory service in the past is also worthwhile.

If indeed the hospital is to provide a comprehensive health care program, it needs to provide adequate discharge planning and follow-up for those patients that need it. In small hospitals, this may occasionally be done by the hospital health educator. More often, a separate discharge planner is available. When such is the case, the hospital health educator and the discharge planner need to work closely together. At a minimum, health education programs available on an outpatient basis need to be made part of the information given during discharge planning. Likewise, the knowledge of community agencies and available programs can be shared by staff in the two programs.

PROGRAMS FOR THE COMMUNITY

The previous chapter discussed self-help programs that might be brought into the hospital and made available to patients and their families. All such

Exhibit 9–1 Health Line

What Is Health Line?

Your direct line by telephone to a tape library of recorded messages which explain special diagnostic tests or procedures. These tests are ordered by doctors to determine a person's state of health.

What is the purpose of Health Line?

. . . to help you understand:

- reasons for test or procedure;
- preparation which may be required;
- procedure to be followed.

How does Health Line work?

- Call 372-5150
- Give the operator the letter and number of the tape you want to hear;
- Listen carefully to the information;
- Call back if you need to hear the tape a second time.

When is Health Line available?

Monday — Friday, 10 a.m. - 9 p.m.; Saturday, 10 a.m. - 6 p.m.

Service is staffed by volunteers in cooperation with the TEL-MED program.

HEALTH LINE
372-5150

Source: Reprinted with permission of Health Education Center, St. Lawrence Hospital, Lansing, Mich., © 1980.

Exhibit 9–1 continued

H-19 Air Colon X-Ray —
x-ray of the colon while expanded with air

H-16 Barium Enema (Colon X-Ray) —
x-ray of part of the large intestine using a special substance

H-63 Blood Culture —
study of blood for disease-producing organisms

H-71 Bone Marrow Aspiration —
removal of the inner soft material of a bone for study

H-52 Bone Scan —
x-ray like picture image of the bones

H-46 Brain Scan —
x-ray like picture image of the brain

H-27 Cardiac Catheterization —
examination of the heart

H-53 Cardiac Scan —
x-ray like picture image of the heart

H-04 Carotid Angiogram (Cerebral) —
x-ray of the neck and head using a special substance

H-07 C.A.T. or E.M.I. Scan —
x-ray like picture image of body portions

H-36 D & C —
ask for Tel-Med tape 74

H-05 E.E.G. (Electroencephalography) —
measure of electrical impulses in the brain

H-26 E.K.G. (Electrocardiogram) —
tracing of electrical activity of the heart

H-06 E.M.G. or N.C.V. (Electromyography) —
measure of electrical impulses in the muscle

H-18 Gallbladder X-Ray —
x-ray of the gallbladder

H-61 Glucose Tolerance Test —
study of blood to measure the body's ability to use sugar

H-41 IVP Infusion (Urinary Exam) —
x-ray of the kidneys, urethra and bladder

H-49 Kidney Scan —
x-ray like picture image of the kidneys

H-21 Liver Biopsy —
removal and examination of liver tissue

H-48 Liver Scan —
x-ray like picture image of the liver

H-51 Lung Scan —
x-ray like picture image of the lungs

H-02 Myelogram —
x-ray of the spinal canal

H-11 Obstetrical Ultrasound —
picture of uterine contents and baby (fetus) in an expectant woman

H-50 Pancreas Scan —
x-ray like picture image of the pancreas

H-22 Paracentesis —
removal of fluid from a body cavity

H-20 Proctoscopy —
visual examination of the rectum

H-32 Pulmonary Function Test (PFT) —
lung performance test

H-01 Spinal Tap (Lumbar Puncture) —
insertion of special needle into spinal canal to obtain fluid

H-62 Sputum Culture —
study of sputum for disease-producing organisms

H-64 Stool Culture —
study of stool for disease-producing organisms

H-31 Thoracentesis —
removal of lung fluids by needle insertion

H-47 Thyroid Scan —
x-ray like picture image of the thyroid

H-17 Upper G.I. (Stomach X-Ray) —
x-ray of stomach, esophagus and duodenum

H-65 Urine Culture —
study of urine for disease-producing organisms

programs can also be provided by the hospital for members of the community as a public relations and health promotion effort.

Some hospitals emphasize their services to the community by providing a health education center. A room or suite of rooms can be made available for classes, support groups, display of literature, etc. Self-instructional programs can also be readily available in learning carrels, and the public can be generally informed that the center is a place to learn about health.

Displays and bulletin boards can be placed in the health education center and throughout the lobbies. Educational materials can also be placed in all waiting rooms. Card files of reprints, pamphlets, etc. can be located there as well, encouraging patients to request specific material that is available either free or on loan.

Regular columns can often be published in area newspapers if medical staff are willing to assist in preparing them. Radio and television spot announcements and talk shows can also be produced and aired when the medical staff, health educators, public relations personnel, and area media cooperate in such programming.

Small hospitals often sponsor "health fairs" with screening for common disorders and educational displays being the primary features. Cosponsorship with the local health department and voluntary agencies spreads the work load, while increasing the number of displays and attendance.

A number of hospitals provide dial-access programs to the community such as Tel Med. Tel Med, a nation-wide program sponsored by Blue Cross and Blue Shield, provides citizens the opportunity to telephone in to hear an audiotape of approximately two minutes in length on a health topic of their choice. The program mandates involvement of the local medical society in cosponsorship with a hospital or other organization. On occasion, Blue Cross and Blue Shield assist the hospital in the initial financing of the project. Major costs involve the facilities (usually donated), the equipment and monthly telephone rates for several lines, staffing (often either switchboard, existing staff, or volunteers), and printing and publicity (often free or donated).

It is also possible to develop tapes locally to add to those available in this program or to use in a similar way, independent of the Tel Med project. One such project is Health Line which explains diagnostic tests or procedures. Whether tests are ordered for inpatients or outpatients, patients can be instructed to dial a number for the needed preparation instructions. Exhibit 9–1 describes one such program.

Many hospitals have closed-circuit television, including production capability. Such hospitals often are located in communities that have cable television and the resultant ability and obligation to program locally. Some hospitals have joined with cable television companies to provide health education programs for the television viewing audience in their community.

CONCLUSION

Hospitals can do as much community health education programming as they have interest and resources. Limited community programs in the past have included weight, stress, and smoking reduction programs; CPR and emergency medical care classes; and patient activation and other self-care classes. Classes or self-instructional modules on specific diseases like diabetes or hypertension were sometimes available. Dial-access systems for audiotapes via telephone or videotapes on closed-circuit or cable television are available only in isolated instances. These programs have been and can be offered independently or brought together in a health education center.

Such programs are wanted, are needed, are judged appropriate by professional associations, and have been tried and found to work. It yet remains to replicate such programs widely and to adequately finance them.

NOTES

1. *Health Education: Role and Responsibility of Health Care Institutions* (Chicago: American Hospital Association, 1975), p. 1.
2. *PROmoting HEALTH* (Chicago: American Hospital Association, 1980).

REFERENCE

Lazes, Peter M., ed. *The Handbook of Health Education.* Rockville, Md.: Aspen Systems Corporation, 1979. (Chapter 2.)

Chapter 10

Funding Health Education Programs

10

INTRODUCTION

As the value of health education is becoming more widely recognized, so the avenues for funding these programs are expanding. With acceptance has come a willingness to invest. Perhaps in the near future that willingness will more fully materialize and bring with it the added dimension of financial stability to health education programs. Yet, in the mean time, securing resources for programs is a major concern for most hospital health educators. Strategies for obtaining such funding is the focus of this chapter.

GENERAL FUNDING STRATEGIES

The problems of funding health education will not simply go away, especially given the runaway health care costs and current efforts at cost containment. While health education contributes to cost containment, it requires the expenditure of money and the passage of time to have the ultimate impact. It costs money to prevent disease as well as to treat disease, though not as much. Unfortunately, many health educators, let alone administrators, do not know how much it costs to prevent disease. Most health educators have not yet attempted to determine the cost per unit of health education. They have operated on the assumption that it should be free, and therefore is free. A beginning strategy for increasing funding is to determine actual costs.[1] It is difficult to get financial support for a service that health educators are unwilling or unable to put a dollar value on. Very few individuals or groups are willing to "write a blank check" for health education.

Administrators and boards are very much concerned with cost containment and struggle with that issue regularly. Accordingly, differing perceptions of health education do affect how the rates are set. It is often necessary to "educate the policy makers" and to work with the fiscal officers to develop the necessary data to do that. A very small change in the rate schedule can often provide a very adequate budget for health education. Administrators and others may need to be reminded of "what is required," "what others are doing," "what the potential is," and "what the public wants." There are good programs that are cost-effective.

A recent survey indicated that 96 percent of the Blue Cross plans and 90 percent of the Blue Shield plans cover patient education when provided as part of treatment. Preventive health education services are covered by 73 percent of the Blue Cross plans and 65 percent of the Blue Shield plans. Costs involved in community health education are covered by 41 percent of the Blue Cross plans and 59 percent of the Blue Shield plans.[2]

If third party payers are not reimbursing for health education costs, it is possible to work collaboratively to change that situation. A professional organization or coalition of organizations could be used effectively to accomplish this change. Third party payers should be approached locally, in writing, to institute changes. Hospital fiscal officers can identify who the appropriate representatives are. It goes without saying that the programs seeking coverage should be of high quality and should include defined target groups, a documentation of need, measurable objectives, appropriate methods for the target group, an evaluation plan, and the credentials of the health educators.

Health educators should also consider the concept of "purchased service" with employees' groups when contracts are being negotiated. Health education and other preventive services are attractive options which may be negotiated into a contract with such an employee group. Health educators may wish to work with fiscal officers in "pricing" such a package and with employee groups in "selling" such a package. Obviously, internal clearance with appropriate administrative staff should be obtained before trying to officially "sell" an employee group any kind of package.

FUNDING PATIENT EDUCATION PROGRAMS

There are three basic ways of financing patient education programs. Each has potential and is being used satisfactorily. Similarly, each has its drawbacks. First, costs may be billed to third party payers in some states. Second, costs may be indirectly carried as part of the daily room rates. The third method is to directly bill patients for educational services rendered. These three methods of financing warrant further exploration, beginning with the most discussed method, third party reimbursement.

Third Party Payer

Third parties in the health care field are insurance companies and government agencies who pay for services that a provider delivers to a consumer. Most often in acute care hospitals, third party reimbursement comes from private insurance companies and the government's Medicaid and Medicare programs.

Third party reimbursement for patient education is considered important because most hospital bills are paid by someone other than the patient. Theoretically, if third party payers are willing to cover health education, ample funds would become available to fund such services. This has already occurred in about a third of the states.

As early as 1974, Blue Cross of America developed a position paper known as the "White Paper on Patient Education." The paper endorsed the concept of patient education, proposed some guidelines, and recommended that several state associations should consider doing likewise. As noted earlier, the Health Insurance Association of America did likewise in 1977. Such coalitions and professional associations, however, are primarily concerned with public relations, and in general, lack implementation capabilities. Implementation must occur at the state level.

Some services currently are routinely covered by third party payers. If the education is directly related to the intake diagnosis and is essential to home care, then reimbursement can occur. If, however, the education deals with other health problems or with prevention in general, reimbursement does not occur under most plans. When such coverage does occur, it is usually simply included in the room and board rates. For example, Medicare's policy states that:

> Reimbursement may be made for such programs to the extent that the programs are appropriate, integral parts in the rendition of covered services which are reasonable and necessary for the treatment of the individual's illness or injury. Where educational activities are not closely related to care and treatment of the patient, such as programs directed toward instructing patients or the public generally in preventive health care activity, reimbursement cannot be made.[3]

It is, therefore, incumbent upon those agencies and institutions wishing reimbursement to bill appropriately. For example, if the visit were for "diabetic follow-up to evaluate injection technique and adherence to diet," it would be more likely to be reimbursed than if it were for diabetic education. Similarly, a visit could be for "amputee follow-up to evaluate gait and prothesis fit," yet include a considerable amount of patient education.[4] This suggestion is not intended to encourage deception, but simply suggests that understanding the reimbursement system and utilizing it properly can enhance the probability of reimbursement. If health educators work closely with the fiscal officer and other administrative personnel, reimbursement can often be found for at least part of a hospital's health education program.

Certainly, the costs of any patient education program will nearly always be passed on to the consumer or the employer who is contributing funds on the employee's behalf. Indeed, such coverage could easily be provided, as with prescription or optical coverage, if an appropriate rider were negotiated and paid for. An educational and lobbying campaign is occurring at present in many states to just this end. Patient education is moving in the direction of wider acceptance as a helpful tool in the medical care process. Future policy revision will likely reflect this trend.

If third party reimbursement for patient education becomes a reality, new problems will emerge. Some patient education specialists view it as a "mixed blessing" at best. One such specialist identified three areas of concern:[5] (1) the potential for waste, (2) a lack of quality control with increased numbers of poorly designed programs, and (3) potential profiteering.

These factors are somewhat interrelated. If programs are poorly designed, inadequately staffed, or inadequately evaluated, there may indeed be great waste. Administrators may spend large sums of money on programs advertised by private companies, sincerely believing the result to be a good program. Such is not necessarily the case.

Concern exists among some patient education specialists, however, that if health education became "revenue producing," many marginal programs would spring into existence. Clearly, standards of practice would have to be agreed upon, and some form of monitoring implemented.

The Health Insurance Association of America spoke to this point when it stated that prior to reimbursement there would need to be:

> (1) acceptance of standards of professional practice, (2) approval of services and programs by the regional Health System's Agencies, and (3) periodic review and approval by the Joint Commission on Accreditation of Hospitals.[6]

While many might question the appropriateness of the HSA's involvement, the philosophy expressed is sound. Quality control is essential to any program, but especially if it is funded by third party reimbursement.

Daily Room Rate

The "indirect costs" mechanism for financing patient education is that by which the health care providers conduct educational programs for patients, but do not separately identify this expenditure on the patient's bill. Such costs are integrated into the patient's "daily room rate" and consequently are indirectly reimbursed by the third party payers.

The daily room rate is not just a flat rate for rental of a room. Actually, the daily room rate includes charges covering many services, such as, (1) three meals-a-day, (2) 24 hour-a-day nursing care, (3) clean sheets and towels, (4) clean and sanitary facilities, and (5) record keeping. Including patient education under this heading is an appropriate way for hospitals to receive reimbursement for a service patients would not receive if identified separately. It is especially appropriate in that patient education has been identified as an integral part of high quality health care.

Most hospitals have quite a low profit margin and often find it difficult to assume the start-up costs and operational expense of a program. However, priorities do come into play. Some hospitals have found discretionary funds to get a program started and have adjusted daily rates to provide for all such services essential to good quality health care. As public policy evolves to demand patient education as part of high quality health care programs, so will acceptance of this method of financing a program.

Adjusting daily room rates to finance patient education is not to be thought of as unethical. This is so especially when one considers that most of the educational activities are carried out by the personnel whose salaries are in fact generated from daily room rates. It is rather an honest, direct attempt to improve total patient care, and as such, should be covered in the daily room rates. This method of financing patient education is working very well in many hospital settings at the present time and seems to be quite practical.

There are, however, certain disadvantages to including the cost of patient education programs in the daily room rates. One, which in fact may seem to be a trivial matter to some, concerns the matter of professionalism. This is a time when health educators are striving to establish themselves as professionals. When their services are not mentioned in the budget of a health care institution, their efforts go, at least partially, unrecognized. This ultimately has an impact on the discipline of health education.

One author describes the problem as follows:

> Health educators often are seen as a "drain" on the budget, a "frill" to be dispensed with in times of tight budgets.

> When patient education becomes a reimbursable item, the health educator (or patient educator) will be viewed as a fiscal asset rather than a liability. This, in turn, will make formal education more available for patients. With additional endeavors justified by patient's needs, will come additional reimbursement. For the health worker this would mean a source of pride and achievement. It would appear more proper to have a separate charge for their services than to have it included with the linen, trash, and cleaning fees of the room charge.[7]

Another potential drawback to this type of funding is that the daily room rates absorb the costs for so many basic and necessary services that it may be difficult to obtain an adequate share for patient education activities when the funds are divided. This may create a dismal picture for the new program, as, for example, when purchasing any extensive educational materials or equipment. It may be hard to justify that one needs new educational equipment when the laundry, garbage, and housekeeping services are all underfunded.

Another disadvantage is the fear that the auditors from the third party payers will uncover these expenses and disallow them. Hospitals have had to pay back large sums of money when this happens. This may, in turn, hamper the relationships between the insurance companies, the hospital administrators, and patient educators, and may also be detrimental to funding future patient education programs. Because of these disadvantages, some programs have chosen to use direct billing of the patient as a means of funding.

Direct Billing

Direct billing is a payment mechanism whereby funds are generated either by directly collecting from the patient receiving the services, or from a separate funding agency or a private source. In most hospitals a fee for each service is usually charged. It may also be appropriate for a fee to be charged for health education. Just because health education has been "free" in the past does not mean it must continue to be in the future. The "hit and miss" efforts of the past may not have required much financing, but it has been established that to do the job right and impact on prognosis and costs, adequate financing is required. Stated differently, free programs are often worth what they charge. Patient education can be billed at the same rates as other clinical services, or even at lower rates, because physicians often are not involved. Where groups are involved, even smaller fees can be charged. The rates should be set to recover actual costs. If staff time is covered in the fixed rates for comprehensive service, it may be appropriate for only an additional charge to be made for educational materials used.

If the patient is to be billed, the patient should have previously agreed to both receive and pay for the educational service. This is usually facilitated by having physicians issue an educational prescription which the patient voluntarily fills, as they would a prescription for medicine. Under this system, it would be the duty of hospital personnel, whether it be the physician, nurse, social worker, patient education coordinator, or whomever, to convince patients it would be for their own well-being to participate in such programs. Patients should not be coerced into a program with direct billing.

The benefits of education are not universally agreed upon, and clients may, therefore, not agree to pay for it. Some patients may refuse to pay simply because they think that knowledge of their illness and how to deal with it should be a part of the routine service provided. This attitude is reflected in the consumer rights' movement.

Hospital administrators will often object to a direct billing program because of the poor public relations it generates. Further, there are extra administrative costs in direct billing. There will also be some bills that will simply not get paid and will have to be written off.

If, however, patient education financing could be successfully handled this way, it would place the discipline of health education on an equal level with other health care providers. Funds could be generated to pay for the services rendered and also to improve those services. It is not, however, considered the most desirable means of program funding.

FUNDING STAFF AND COMMUNITY PROGRAMS

Staff and community programs are often small programs that are simply an integral part of the larger patient education programs funded as discussed above. However, when staff and community programs are larger, very visible efforts, separate funding mechanisms must often be established.

In the past, such projects have been funded as pilot projects by grants or endowments. There are still limited funds available for such purposes, but they are not adequate to finance all the needed programs.

The division of Special Operations of the Bureau of Health Insurance (BHI) has funded pilot programs to evaluate health education's potential for cost effectiveness. Selected programs which meet the requirements of P.L. 92–603 for experiments in reimbursement may be funded on an experimental basis, even though they involve prevention. Likewise, the BHI has limited funds available for pilot programs. Perhaps more importantly, this agency monitors availability of funds from other sources and can advise those seeking funding on currently available sources. The Department of Agriculture is involved in financing rural health education programs that work with the Cooperative Extension Service. Another possible source of funding is the National Health Service Corporation. A recent survey[8] found that 93 percent of the Blue Cross or Blue Shield programs are also financing innovative health education programs to document the cost effectiveness of life style modification and illness prevention.

Anyone who is going to seek external funding should work closely with an agency grantswriter or someone who has had grant writing experience. The following list of "dos" is a concise summary of the basics:[9]

- Obtain internal approval. Get it as part of the agency's priority list.
- Establish reasonable goals. Establish a good evaluation procedure to help measure impact.
- Identify potential prospects, preferably in the locale. *The Foundation Directory* can be of assistance in this matter.
- Get internal clearance before approaching personnel of any funding source. Other members of your staff could conceivably be working with that same group on a project that is more important to your agency.
- Make an initial approach with a letter of inquiry, a summary of your idea, and a promise to call.
- Set-up an informal meeting and make your presentation. Be positive. Discuss the idea and get suggestions.
- Write the formal proposal. Get appropriate signatures. Present it formally.
- Say "thank you" for their contribution or their consideration.

Again, proposals should be presented initially at the local level and should contain at minimum a definition of the target group, a documented need, measurable objectives, appropriate methods, an evaluation plan, and the credentials of the director with an adequate explanation of why the program is important.

Local or area funding sources should not be overlooked. These include but are not limited to voluntary health agencies, industries, retired health care professionals, churches, service clubs, etc. Sometimes such agencies will cosponsor a hospital-based program that meets a need they are also interested in, and they will share the costs.

A relatively new method of financing that appears to have promise is to package and sell health promotion programs to groups or businesses in the area. Hospitals often have the expertise, facilities, and credibility to develop employee assistance programs and other health promotion programs to meet the increasing needs of area industries. Certainly health promotion programs developed for hospital staff may be marketable to other groups in the area, at a profit, which then can often be used for other health education programs.

CONCLUSION

Cost containment is not a concept that applies to everyone else; it can and should apply to health educators as well. Health educators should continually be looking for ways to "keep the costs down" and to get more results with the same money.

Health educators should be looking for free or inexpensive materials to use in their programs. They should be using resource people from community agencies. Sharing of health educators also has potential, in that expertise and programs available in one agency can be traded for expertise and programs currently available in another. Obviously, a good working relationship is required between the two health educators and the other staff involved. Also of importance is to be certain that the program is localized so as to be appropriate to the new target group.

Programs that are currently operating one-on-one can perhaps be expanded to a group setting so as to be more cost-efficient. Programs using high salaried staff can often use low salaried staff effectively with sufficient planning. Effective management of the health education program will take all these factors into consideration and will often end up with a combination of staff members all used effectively.

A high priced program that prevents disease or disorders is cost-efficient, but a lower priced program may be more effective and, therefore, more cost-effective. Expensive programs aren't always the best, and certainly aren't always the most cost-efficient. Likewise, the most inexpensive programs aren't always the best or the most cost-effective.

Good managers will have their primary focus on program effectiveness continually monitoring the program to seek ways of improvement. Such formative data can and should be considered within the context of cost containment; i.e., can the program be as effective using less expensive materials, methods, or staff? But in the final analysis, the emphasis has to be on effectiveness, program quality, and evaluation data that helps managers determine if the program is working. Only then can good decisions be made relative to whether the impact is worth the cost.

There are ways to finance good health education programs. Literally hundreds of programs are currently in existence. Existing programs were implemented because of an adminstrative commitment to the concept. Institutions with an annual budget often exceeding a million dollars can find money for a health program if there is serious commitment. Institutional priorities have to be established regarding expenditure of funds. While it is true that there is rarely enough funds for everything an institution wishes to do, it is also true that educational programs have often been very low on the list of priorities, and have in reality, often been given only "lip service." Fortunately, this situation is changing rapidly.

NOTES

1. Sue Pritchett, *Financing Patient and Family Education at the Hospital Level* (Chicago: National Conference on Hospital-Based Patient Education, 1976), p. 5
2. *Survey Report, Blue Cross and Blue Shield Plan Support for Health Education* (Chicago: Blue Cross/Blue Shield, 1979), p. 11.
3. *Reimbursement Forum Proceedings* (Chicago: American Hospital Association, 1979), p. 119.
4. Susan Pritchett, *Financing Patient and Family Education*, p. 5.
5. Scott Simonds, "Third Party Reimbursement for Patient Education Services: What's Happening and Why Not," Speech delivered before the Society for Public Health Education, Great Lakes Chapter (Lansing, Mi.: Michigan Department of Public Health, 1978).
6. *Financing In Hospital Patient Education* (New York: Health Insurance Association of America, 1977), p. 3.
7. Beatrice Nordberg and Lynelle King, "Third Party Payment for Patient Education," *American Journal of Nursing*, August 1976, p. 1271.
8. *Survey Report, Blue Cross and Blue Shield Plan Support for Health Education*, p. 11.
9. *PROmoting HEALTH* (Chicago: American Hospital Association, March-April 1980), pp. 1–3.

Chapter 11

Record Keeping and Program Evaluation

11

INTRODUCTION

All hospital programs must keep records, and health education programs are not exempt from this requirement. Utilized primarily in program evaluation, as will be discussed later in this chapter, records also have direct impact on any liability suits that are initiated. Liability suits are more probable when educating patients than when educating staff or members of the community.

LEGAL CONSIDERATIONS

Liability is of concern to most people who work in and around a hospital. However, if some basic procedures are followed, it need not get in the way of establishing and maintaining a good program. Indeed, it can lead to a better educational program, because it usually causes educators to teach units as they were intended to be taught.

Liability is based on negligence. While anyone can sue, a liability judgment is based on established negligence. Negligence is based in large part on what a reasonably prudent person would do, or in this situation, what a reasonably prudent health educator would do.

All hospital employees should carry some form of liability insurance coverage. The hospital may have a blanket policy covering all employees, which should be investigated as to availability and adequacy. In its absence, professional associations often offer low cost liability insurance to members of their group. A third option is to work with a private insurance carrier to add a liability rider to existing coverage.

One item of special concern should be noted. Insurance does not always cover the cost of legal defense. With the quickness to sue that seemingly exists, such coverage by the hospital or in a personal insurance package seems appropriate.

Reasonably prudent hospital health educators use well-planned programs and carefully selected materials. They assess patient's needs and provide appropriate programs. They also keep records of what they have done and at least their perceptions of what they have accomplished.

BASIC CONSIDERATIONS IN RECORD KEEPING

Patients' records are a written account of what happens to them while in the medical care system. Records are admissable in court, can be subpoenaed, and often have a major impact on the outcome of a case. They should be accurate and complete. Entries should be made when an event occurs and should be dated and signed. They should never be erased, even if incorrect, because erasures may give the appearance of trying to hide something. Instead, inaccurate entries should have a line drawn through them and an explanatory note entered, dated, and signed.

Records should be kept as long as the "statute of limitations" is in effect, which varies from state to state. Records for minors should normally be kept for a corresponding length of time after the minor becomes legally an adult. Patients sometimes bring suit for injuries sustained by them when they were minors.

Records should be factual and written from the vantage point of the professional making an entry on the record. There may be legitimately different perceptions, which if entered, must again be signed and dated.

The record is the legal property of the hospital, but patients and their approved representatives usually have access to it, if need be by court order. Patients can give written authorization to release their records to insurance companies, worker compensation programs, pension programs, and others who have a legitimate interest in the case.

While much of the discussion of this chapter has been and will be on legal implications, there is an even more basic use that ought to be in the forefront of any decisions on record keeping. A patient's record is an instrument that is used in planning care and individualizing the treatment regimen. It is used to remind staff quickly and accurately of the patient's history, diagnosis, and prescribed regimen. It is the chief means of communication among the staff on the three shifts and the many departments of a hospital that may be involved in a patient's treatment program. The first and foremost consideration should, therefore, be to record data that will assist those caring for the patient to make the best decisions possible. However, experience has taught those in the health care field that all such decisions must be made within the context of possible litigation at some unspecified future time.

There are two basic types of medical records. The older and more traditionally used record is a chronological recording of significant events. The newer procedure is a "problem oriented medical record." In the "POMR" process, a list of problems the patient has is kept current in the front of the chart. Each problem so specified requires that a plan be developed to alleviate the problem. The plan may involve more diagnostic work, therapy, or education. Notes regarding progress are numbered and titled to correspond to the problem list in the front of the chart. The problem oriented medical record is generally preferred by patient educators since it helps practitioners see health education as part of the solution to patient problems.

Either approach can be used effectively in a patient education program. Hospital health educators must first of all ascertain what type of record keeping is currently being used in the institution. They must then decide how patient education can best fit into that system or how record keeping can be modified to incorporate the needs of health education.

Hospital health education personnel will usually also develop records of their own, which will not be entered into a patient's primary chart. It is common for educational notes to be entered in the patient's primary record and for a supplementary set of records be kept in the education department. This also has the effect of keeping the medical record or chart less bulky. Educational personnel should follow all the basic considerations listed above in record keeping, even though the records are kept in the education department.

EDUCATIONAL RECORDS

A variety of educational records may be kept, but the first such form should usually be a referral form. This form is especially important if there is to be billing specifically for the educational program. The form may or may not have diagnostic or prescription elements built into it. It may indeed be called an educational prescription.

There are two major ways commonly used in which a patient can be referred to the health education program. The preferred method is by the use of "standing orders." It is possible to work with the medical staff when developing the program or to review it with them in sufficient detail so that they are comfortable in referring all patients with that diagnosis. For example, all diabetic patients could be routinely seen by the health education staff and assessed for educational needs. If such a blanket approval was obtained from the staff as a whole or from individual physicians, more patients would get involved in the educational program. A well-developed program and a cooperative relationship with the medical staff are usually required before the referral becomes automatic.

In the absence of standing orders, a printed referral slip can be attached to the chart of appropriate patients for the physician to sign. Such an "educational prescription" can be to the program in its entirety or to a specific component of it. The educational protocol can be built into the referral form in checklist fashion, so as to facilitate use, as in Exhibit 11–1.

As will be discussed in Chapter 14, there is also a need to perform an educational needs assessment for each patient seen. If an intake interview is done by education staff, it too should be included in the patient's records.

It is important to document what has been taught to patients and their families and to document whether or not comprehension or competency has been demonstrated. Comprehension or competency can be demonstrated by observing the patient, as for example in the use of equipment

Exhibit 11–1 Patient Education Order Form

Patient's name ______________________ Chart # __________
If currently an outpatient:
Address ______________________________________
______________________ Telephone __________
This patient should be enrolled in the following education program(s):
_ The entire diabetic education program or the following specific sessions
 _ Diabetes: What it is and how to live with it?
 _ Diabetic diet
 _ Diabetic medications
 _ Urine testing
 _ Diabetic emergencies
_ This patient should not be enrolled in the diabetic education program
Comments:

Signed ______________________ Date __________

Note: This form should be sent to the Education Department of Community Hospital when completed.

by the chronic obstructive pulmonary disease patient. Discussion with the patient also provides the staff with the opportunity to at least have patients describe their understandings. Such ability to verbalize is not definitive. It is, however, a baseline indication of comprehension or competency for which a reasonably prudent patient educator should strive. The column indicating understanding should only be dated and signed when comprehension or competency has been demonstrated in some way. In court cases, records may be subpoenaed, and it is essential to the outcome of some cases to have such records available.

As was discussed in previous chapters, major concepts can be briefly cataloged, and columns established for dates and signatures. The listing helps ensure that a comprehensive program has at least been considered. The concepts need not be preprinted, however. The patient educator can enter whatever concepts are actually taught. Exhibit 11–2 is an example of one approach.

PROGRAM EVALUATION PROCEDURES*

Evaluation conjures up to many images of computers, reams of paperwork, and complicated statistical formulas. These are often thought to be unmanagable and beyond the scope of educators. As a result, too many educators don't attempt any formal means of evaluation.

There are other reasons besides lack of experience and expertise why people do not evaluate their programs. One reason is a fear that the evaluation results will be unfavorable and might force changes with "the way things are done." Yet another obstacle to evaluation is scarce resources. It takes time and money to do program evaluation, both of which are often severely limited. It is easy to decide consciously or subconsciously not to evaluate a program, or more commonly, to decide that evaluation is something that will be done later.

Sometimes evaluation is done with sophisticated statistical analysis using computers and research consultants. This evaluation may show areas in the program where improvements can be made. Planners need not be defensive about such results, since virtually all programs can be improved with added staff time and increased fiscal resources for program analysis. However, program evaluation can be done just as effectively and far less expensively with existing program staff. The focus of this section will be

*This section based on Donald J. Breckon and Sherrie LeClear, "Does Patient Education Help Anyone?" by permission of *Michigan Health Educator,* © August 1980.

Exhibit 11–2 Patient Education Record

Patient's name ______________________ Chart # __________

Address ____

______________________________ Telephone __________

Patient education program ______________________________

	Patient			Family		
	Initial instruction	Review and reinforcement	Demonstrates compliance	Initial instruction	Review and reinforcement	Demonstrates compliance
Concept Medical regimen Side effects to be reported Low sodium diet etc.						

__ Educational material given to patient (please specify)
__ Invited to attend the program again as an outpatient
__ Referred to community educational program (please specify)

on how to plan and implement a satisfactory evaluation using resources immediately at hand.

Rationale

There are two major types of evaluation. *Formative evaluation* is usually the first phase and attempts to assess how well the program is going. It is sometimes called process evaluation. It is used throughout a project and provides data that will help improve a program. It includes some of the needs assessment discussed earlier, the pretesting of material, and the general assessment of efficiency.

The primary purpose of formative evaluation efforts is to improve the program as it continues. Such evaluation helps determine whether the program is moving in the right direction, and whether the goals are being met. It may or may not include analysis to be used to gain support for program expansion. It may also be used to compare the relative effectiveness of different approaches to the same problem and to support program revision.

Summative evaluation on the other hand is more concerned with measuring the impact of a program. It usually focuses on determining if the goals and objectives of the program have been met and at what cost. It is usually done at the conclusion of a program or at specified intervals, for example, annually.

Summative evaluation is an attempt to demonstrate that a program is worthwhile and to justify the expenditure of time and energy. Such evaluation is usually required for funding sources, board members, and administrative superiors. Even if supervisory boards and staff do not demand such documentation, it is usually appreciated. An employee's stature as a program director will be enhanced because of such efforts.

Evaluation data can also be used as a public relations tool, improving the image of the program with other hospital staff and with the community. Evaluation reports are usually newsworthy and are of interest to local media.

Another important use of evaluation studies is to publish them in journals so that colleagues can learn from them. Such reports can be useful to others initiating or administering similar programs. Comparisons can be beneficial if comparable data is available.

Program evaluation is now considered an essential part of program planning and implementation. It does have payoffs, since client, staff, program, and administrator all stand to gain.

The Basics

An evaluation component should start with specific program objectives that spell out in measurable terms what outcomes are desirable. It is of utmost importance when planning a program to write objectives in such a way that data can be gathered to measure if the objective has been met. For example, one objective might read, "At least 80% of the hypertensive patients will be within 10% of their recommended weight within six months."

If the originator of a program did not spell out objectives in such a way, the first step in planning an evaluation component is to write measurable objectives. Then, depending on the objectives, data needs to be gathered to measure whether the objectives have been met.

The degree of sophistication used in the evaluation scheme will sometimes be determined by the funding source. When such guidelines occur, they must obviously be followed completely. In the absence of such guidelines, the following three factors ought to be considered:

1. *Effort.* It is always important to determine how much effort is expended on the program. At minimum, a record keeping system ought to be developed that would keep track of the number of clients entering and/or completing a program. A breakdown by age and sex, at the least, may be helpful. It often is also helpful to determine the source of referrals to the program.

   If various program time slots are used, future planning would be well-served by recording attendance at the various time frames. If various educational formats are offered, the frequency of which the format is chosen should be recorded. If the health educator has other job responsibilities, the number of hours spent actually doing health education ought to be recorded.

   These measures of effort are often revealing in and of themselves. Very often, educational staff and their supervisors will be unaware of how great their effort is until accounting occurs. Also, a measurement of effort is basic to other evaluation techniques.
2. *Efficiency.* It is always important to evaluate the administration of a program and to examine typical procedures for efficiency. A staff meeting should be held, at least annually, specifically to examine problem areas and to suggest ways of doing the necessary tasks more efficiently without a decrease in quality.

   A written report should be prepared and distributed and the results implemented. About every fifth year an external review of the program can be conducted using appropriate consultants from other hospitals, professional societies, and college or university personnel. Far more elaborate studies can be done, such as cost-effectiveness studies, but they usually require expert help and technical equipment to utilize.
3. *Effectiveness.* It is theoretically possible to expend a lot of effort and not accomplish very much. Effort is a prerequisite, but certainly not a guarantee of impact. While it is extremely difficult to prove that there has been an impact on a client, it is feasible to gather evidence that suggests that there has been an impact. Such measures should be immediate, and, if time and resources permit, long-term.

   Immediate evaluation of effectiveness should include feed-back from clients and staff focusing on perceived appropriateness and effectiveness. Simple, one-page checklists can be developed. Hand-tallying can be used if a numerical value is placed on each response. A five-point Lickert Scale is typical. Highly Satisfied—5, Somewhat Satisfied—4, Neutral—3, Somewhat Dissatisfied—2, and Highly Dissatisfied—1. It can easily be a three point scale, based simply on satisfactory, neutral, or unsatisfactory. Scores can easily be computed for each client or staff member as well as for groups of clients or staff. New programs ought to administer such checklists to all clients and staff members during the first six months of the program. Insights gained ought to be fed back into the program via revisions, and again evaluated. Such a feed-back loop ought always to exist. Large programs can be revised and evaluated every three months. Small programs should wait six months or a year until sufficient data has been collected on which to base a decision. As the program matures and stabilizes, the time frame being evaluated ought to lengthen so that the time demanded for evaluation can be kept reasonable.

Long-range impact is more time-consuming to measure. Interviews via telephone or home visits are needed to measure selected impact indicators. The indicators chosen will vary for specific diseases, but will include factors, such as, compliance with physician's orders, ability to handle emergencies that arise, and readmission rates. Random samples can be selected every third year for such study.

CONCLUSION

Record keeping is an important element in any health education program. There are many varieties of records and no imperative exists for all programs to use the same format. There is, however, good reason to use standard record keeping procedures. Prevention is the key to many liability judgments. The availability of accurate records is often the major determinant of the outcome of a legal case.

Records are also an integral part of program evaluation, used to measure the effectiveness of an offering. Data gathered in this fashion is not absolutely valid, that is, it doesn't necessarily prove that the effect measured was a direct result of the program. Many other variables may intervene which should be controlled where possible. It does, however, provide a sounder basis on which to plan for the future than if the evaluation had not occurred. A great deal can be learned about what works and what doesn't, even though it cannot be proven beyond a shadow of a doubt.

To refuse to perform program evaluation because "it doesn't prove anything" is counterproductive. Those who desire to improve the effectiveness and efficiency of their programs will evaluate them and as a result will find both efficiency and effectiveness spiraling upwards.

REFERENCES

Anderson, Scarvia B.; Ball, Samuel; and Murphy, Richard T. *Encyclopedia of Educational Evaluation.* San Francisco: Jossey Bass, 1977.

Anderson, Scarvia B. and Ball, Samuel. *The Profession and Practice of Program Evaluation.* San Francisco: Jossey Bass, 1978.

Fink, Arlene. *An Evaluation Primer.* Washington, D.C.: Capitol Publications, 1977.

Schulberg, Herbert C. *Program Evaluation in the Health Fields.* New York: Behavioral Publications, 1979.

Part III

Health Education Practice

part III

The preceding section has focused on the administrative aspects of planning, implementing, and evaluating a program. It detailed the tasks of the director, coordinator, or administrator of the health education program. Part III assumes that an educational policy has been developed, staff have been selected and trained, a needs assessment has been performed, and needed curricula are in place, or are at least in the process of being developed. Programs are at the teaching and learning stage. Good teaching can overcome the absence of appropriately developed program elements; conversely, poor teaching can negate the impact of a carefully designed program. Accordingly, it is important to concentrate more on the educational dimensions of programming than on administrative tasks. The focus of this section, then, is on the tasks of the health educator, patient instructor, or others actually involved in teaching the client.

Chapter 12

An Introduction to the Theoretical Foundations of Hospital Health Education

12

INTRODUCTION

Health education is usually concerned with behavior change, regardless of the educational setting in which it takes place or the group that is targeted. However, it should be noted that health education is not concerned with change at any cost or change by any methods. Certainly the use of force is ruled out in favor of persuasion. Likewise, various methods of manipulating behavior are usually considered inappropriate. The brainwashing techniques used on prisoners of wars or by cults are likewise considered out of place. Even behavior modification is suspect, if indeed, the client is not involved in the decision to modify behavior.

This author's philosophical basis for hospital health education programs, then, is that of "informed decision making." This concept is emphasized in the definition in the Michigan Public Health Code.

> Health education is that dimension of health care that directs attention of individuals to their health behavior with the goal of enabling them to make reasoned decisions about their own health practices and those within the various communities in which they live and work and play. The basic components of reasoned health decision making education include both (a) the acquisition of accurate, unbiased, authoritative knowledge of subjects such as human biology, efficacy of early prevention, disease detection and control, alternative health practices and the consequences of each, and the effective assessment of an individual's own beliefs on health outcomes and, (b) The acquisition of behavior skills required to carry out the desired alternative.[1]

As a result of such an educational process, the clients should be able to make informed decisions that are appropriate for them. The client's decision should be a better decision after considering the alternatives, weighing the consequences of alternative actions, and deciding on an appropriate course of action, with of course, staff input. But it should be clear to all concerned, that the final decision, to participate or not and to comply or not, is that of the client, unless, of course, the client is a minor or is too ill to make the necessary decisions.

ANDRAGOGICAL APPROACH

Andragogy is the theory and practice of educating adults, as contrasted to pedagogy which is concerned with the education of children. Inasmuch as most of the clients in a hospital health education program will be adults, theoretical foundations must include an understanding of the principles of educating adults. This is essential from a practical point of view since most adults have had more experience being taught as a child and tend to teach as they were taught. While it is often appropriate to treat children as if they were adults, it is seldom appropriate to treat adults as if they were children when they are involved in the educational enterprise.

When entering into a discussion of this nature, staff need to remember the many ways that adults are different from children. Obviously, adults are physically mature and legally responsible for their behavior. But far more important to the educational process, adults have a more definite mind-set than children. Their likes and dislikes are more fixed and their attitudes are more difficult to change. Their feelings about authority are more likely to be negative, because they now consider themselves to be independent and self-directing. They are less likely to do what they are told and must see the relevance of what is being proposed quite quickly, or the instruction is apt to be ignored.

Adults are capable of learning a great deal, but are often unwilling to exert effort to learn that which does not meet a need for them. Adults are capable of learning at all ages as well. The rate at which learning occurs slows down somewhat as physiological changes occur during the aging process, but the ability to learn is there unless destroyed by disease or disorders.[2]

The key to adult education, then, is helping adults see the relevance of what they need to know, so that in their self-directing way, they will choose to learn about regaining or maintaining their health. Stated differently, the central purpose of health education is to bring valid knowledge to bear on the decisions that clients must make. In so doing, it is aimed at achieving the needs and goals that the individual specifies, and if possible, to also satisfy the needs and goals of the hospital and society. The importance of a needs assessment becomes instantly apparent to those subscribing to this approach.

Health education of adults should also be situation-oriented rather than subject-oriented, in order to make the relevance of it obvious and to maintain interest. Too much instruction can be as bad as none. It is not necessary to tell patients everything that might be useful. If health education focuses on present or future situations that clients will probably encounter, interest is usually easy to maintain. Other problems can be dealt with if and when they occur. Health education should be an encounter with reality. It should involve coming to grips with the world in which learners find themselves. Their new knowledge should help learners in the process of understanding and interpreting whatever they encounter.[3]

Effective Teaching Principles

The following principles of effective curricula development and teaching in adult education programs are adapted from the basic work *The Modern Practice of Adult Education: Andragogy versus Pedagogy.*[4]

1. Begin with a need assessment of the client or clients. It is critical to interest and motivation that learners feel a need to learn, and that they make that decision to learn because they see a need for it. It is important to respect adult clients as self-directing human beings.

An accompanying staff role is to expose learners to new possibilities, presenting what they need to learn in order to adequately confront current or future problems. Other significant staff roles are to assist learners to diagnose their learning needs, and then to decide what is to be learned and how it is to be learned. Such a cooperative relationship requires trust, which leads to the second principle.

2. Establish a learning environment that is characterized by physical comfort, mutual trust, and freedom of expression. Having an adequate physical environment is basic, yet often difficult to obtain in a hospital. Whenever possible, facilities should be available that have adequate lighting, heating, and ventilation; flexible seating; and adequate audio-visual capabilities. Whenever there are interruptions, distractions, noises, uncomfortable temperature or humidity, or inadequate lighting, attention is distracted away from learning.

Of even more importance, however, is the development of an emotional climate that facilitates learning. This starts with the basics of establishing rapport and accepting and respecting each person as an individual of worth with his or her own feelings and ideas. It includes establishing an atmosphere of mutual responsibility whenever possible, so that clients and staff are learning from each other.

3. Involve the client as much as possible in the learning process. As mentioned earlier, learners need to be assisted in setting their own learning goals and selecting learning experiences from those available to them. The educator should also help clients exploit the experience of both themselves and others while learning. The experience that adults bring to a learning encounter is another major difference between adults and children. Those who would teach adults effectively must learn to use these experiences effectively.

The client must also be involved in the learning process as much as possible so as to maximize learning. Active learning is preferable to passive learning. If students are involved in thinking, discussing, viewing, trying, etc., learning is more apt to take place. The more of the five senses that can be involved in the learning, the more learning will occur.

4. Learners must be kept apprized of their progress toward their goals. The educator can do this in part by facilitating self-evaluation on the part of the learners, or can monitor progress and report it as perceived by the staff. Such feed-back is important. Pacing is also important. If teaching is faster or slower than individual readiness, learning will be inhibited.

Another role in this process is to assist learners in rediagnosis, that is, an assessment of what has already been learned and of what yet needs to be learned. Thus, the process is cyclical, and should ideally lead to life-long learning.

Self-Directed Learning

Concurrently, learners must also be made aware of resources for self-directed study. Because interest and motivation is usually high, referrals to books, pamphlets, community classes, etc. will often be followed. Such self-directed learning is facilitated by awareness of and ready availability of resources.

Alan Tough in his works indicates that self-directed learning is most probable when there is interest in inquiry, a sense of optimism, an adequate energy level, and a sense of power or control over life situations.[5] Accordingly, health educators working with adults should stimulate a sense of inquiry and encourage a sense of optimism and control. Certainly there is the potential for learning about health to be life-long. There is also the potential for far more learning to occur outside the formal learning experience than in it. Adult educators should encourage self-directed learning.

APPROACHES TO BEHAVIOR CHANGE

It has been established through research that people generally go through several stages before changing a behavior. These stages come in a more or less logical sequence, albeit at differing rates. These steps are described with variations, but usually involve (1) awareness of the proposed change, (2) interest in it, (3) trial, and (4) adoption of the new behavior. Educators who would facilitate adult learning should begin by assessing the stage where the majority of their learners are. If most learners are at the stage of developing awareness and interest, then differing educational techniques are appropriate than if the need is for trial or adoption of the recommended practice.

Creating awareness and interest on a large scale can be effectively done via mass media. Getting people to try a procedure and continue doing it is obviously more difficult, and most generally requires more personalized, face-to-face attention. While posters, displays, pamphlets, or other spot announcements may publicize a program and create interest in it, such approaches will not usually create trial and adoption. Conversely, there is little need to spend time, energy, and money creating interest in a subject if that interest is already present.

Educators who work for behavior change in their clients need also to pay considerable attention to reinforcing the decisions to try or adopt a recommended health practice. Many people have tried to lose weight or stop smoking, but have been unsuccessful in their attempts. Personal and group effort to reinforce good decisions are needed. Much of the success of Alcoholics Anonymous and other such programs may be related to the fact that their programs offer personal support systems where progress is monitored and clients are reinforced when needed. The weekly meetings and telephone hot lines of other programs are also helpful. The personal interest and peer pressure of people in a support group including, but not limited to, staff is also helpful in the adoption process.

Knowledge alone is usually not enough to get desirable behavior change. Few people follow all the good health practices they know they ought to do. As discussed earlier, it is, therefore, important to plan educational activities that get at attitudes within the affective domain. It cannot be safely assumed that a change in knowledge will result in a change in attitude which will then result in a change in behavior. Such change needs to be programmed at all three stages.

Beliefs Model

One approach to getting at the affective dimension of behavior change has been described in a large body of research, known as the Beliefs Model,[6] which assumes that what people believe is as important as what they know. The Beliefs Model focuses on perceptions of susceptibility, severity, benefits, and barriers. It shows that these perceptions or beliefs are more influential than the actual degree of susceptibility, severity, benefits, and barriers. For example, if a client felt highly susceptible to a severe disorder, then that client would probably act if there was a preventive behavior that was perceived to be effective in reducing the risk. Conversely, people at high risk that don't perceive that risk are unlikely to take preventive action.

Health educators with this philosophical orientation can incorporate elements of this model in their educational activities when possible. When planning lectures, discussions, counseling sessions, designing literature, etc., they can include content or methods that will impart a sense of susceptibility to consequences that are perceived by the client to be severe. Also, they can call attention to how the recommended behavior will help reduce those risks. If the benefits of engaging in that risk reduction behavior outweigh the barriers, most clients will adopt the recommended behavior. Providing cues or triggers to precipitate the desired behavior change is also appropriate.

Consider a diabetic patient. Such a patient needs to be aware of his/her susceptibility to diabetic coma and the serious nature of this disorder once onset has occurred. The educator can recommend behaviors including regulation of food, exercise, and medicine that are relatively easy to do, so that the benefits outweigh the barriers to the recommended action. Most clients that go through such a session will adopt the proposed behavior changes. Such a process can be applied to any behavior change that is needed in a patient's therapy.

A note of caution should be added about unduly arousing high levels of fear and anxiety. Fear can stimulate interest, but is not usually the basis for sustained behavior change. A realistic assessment of the risks involved is appropriate. Educators should, however, avoid the temptation to exaggerate by taking the worst possible case and portraying it as typical, or their credibility is at stake.

Value Clarification

The use of value clarification exercises hold considerable promise for health education. As the title suggests, they are a series of exercises designed to help people clarify what they value and what that value means to their behavior. Such techniques have been widely used in the public schools, but have potential for health education in hospital settings as well. They are also consistent with the andragogical approach to health education. When working with children, it is more typical to transmit values from a position of experience or authority. When working with adults, it is preferable to help them clarify their own values. The exercises themselves are intended to be thought provoking, and often are useful ways to move quickly to meaningful discussion on sensitive topics. Those interested in using these techniques are urged to enroll in a class or workshop on the topic.

Behavior Modification

Behavior modification was mentioned briefly in the early part of this chapter. This concept can be used effectively in a hospital setting with, as specified earlier, the clients consent. Behavior modification techniques are being effectively used in weight control and in stop smoking programs. There is potential to adapt the principles to other aspects of health education. As with value clarification, a discussion of the procedure in detail is outside the scope of this book. References are suggested for those who wish to study these techniques. College courses are also available in many places.

PRECEDE Model

Another part of the theoretical approach to hospital health education is in Green's PRECEDE Model.[7] PRECEDE is an acronym for predisposing, reinforcing, and enabling causes in educational diagnoses and evaluation. Predisposing factors refer to the knowledge, attitudes, and values that a person brings to a decision and have been previously discussed in other contexts. Enabling factors are the principal new item not discussed earlier in this book, and refer to availability and accessibility of resources. People simply aren't able to do what is best for their health on all occasions. Work with the family, the hospital, social worker, or community agencies is often necessary. The model postulates that when a person is predisposed to act, enabled to act, and reinforced for that action, behavior change will occur. Health educators would be well-advised to focus elements of the educational process on these three facets of the model. As mentioned earlier, it is also important to do an educational diagnosis to ascertain need and to evaluate any education delivered.

CONCLUSION

Theory and practice have been contrasted for years. It has also been said that there is nothing so practical as a good theory.

Health behavior is complex, with multiple causes and consequences. Rarely is a single theory sufficient to explain a situation. Yet an understanding of appropriate theories and application of them to learning situations will enhance the probability that learning will occur and that the desired behavior will subsequently evolve.

Regardless of the theories or methods used, teaching will not have the desired impact in all cases. Some prospective learners simply will not respond. Others will respond, but long after they leave the hospital. While it is important to evaluate the effectiveness of programs, remember that those successes that are reported will represent minimal achievement. Unaccounted for are those who find that learning is reinforced at a later time and who respond at an appropriate time. However, using sound educational theory does increase the probability of having the effect that is desired.

NOTES

1. Michigan Public Health Code, Section 2237.
2. T. W. Elwood, "Relationship of Health Education to Gerontology," *International Journal of Health Education* 15 (1972): 3–19.
3. Russell Kleis, *Basic Propositions With Respect to Adult and Continuing Education* (East Lansing, Mi.: Michigan State University, 1979), p.1.
4. Malcolm Knowles, *The Modern Practice of Adult Education* (New York: Association Press, 1973), p. 384.
5. Alan Tough, *The Adults Learning Projects* (Toronto: Ontario Institute for Studies in Education, 1971), p. 192.
6. Irwin Rosenstock, *Implications of the Health Belief Model for Educational Practice* (Ann Arbor, Mi.: University of Michigan Course Handout, 1975) p. 2.
7. Lawrence Green et al., *Health Education Planning: A Diagnostic Approach* (Palo Alto, Ca.: Mayfield Publishing Co., 1980), p. 306.

REFERENCES

Cross, K. Patricia. *Adults as Learners.* San Francisco: Jossey Bass, 1981.

Houle, Cyril. *Continuing Learning in the Professions.* San Francisco: Jossey Bass, 1980.

Knowles, Malcolm S. *The Modern Practice of Adult Education: Andragogy vs. Pedagogy.* Chicago: Association Press, 1980.

Knox, Alan B. *Adult Development and Learning.* San Francisco: Jossey Bass, 1977.

Ross, Helen S. and Mico, Paul R. *Theory and Practice of Health Education.* Palo Alto, Ca.: Mayfield Publishing Co., 1980.

Chapter 13

Communication and Motivation: The Essence of Health Education

13

INTRODUCTION

All the good theories, good content, good methods, and good materials in the world will not assure that health education is taking place unless there are two elements present: communication and motivation. While elements of these topics have been touched on earlier, a discussion of them in more detail is important to those engaged in the practice of health education.

COMMUNICATION

Communication is central to the education process. It can be either written or oral, and health educators need to be effective at both.

The burden of communication is usually on the person responsible for doing the teaching. Therefore, such dissemination of concepts should be carefully planned so as to enhance the probability that a message is acutally received and used. One useful way of looking at the communication process is through the model shown in Figure 13–1.

Figure 13–1 Communication Process

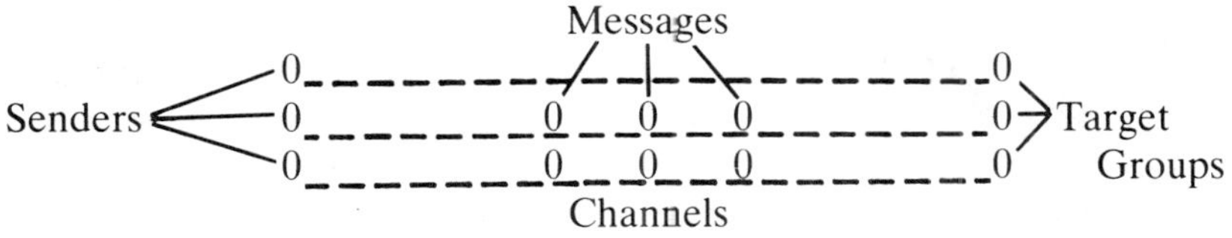

As mentioned in earlier chapters, the target group to be educated should be carefully selected to be homogeneous and as narrowly defined as possible. This usually results in there being more than one target group in a program. Pragmatically, it often means adapting a given program to more than one group.

The educational messages needed should then be identified. Once the group and the messages have been identified, the most effective senders and channels should be selected to deliver the messages to the target group, and a process of feed-back implemented to be sure that the message is received.

A given educational program will often involve several target groups. It may be necessary to reach the patient, those caring for the patient, and personnel in community agencies. Different messages may be appropriate for the differing groups, though all may need some common information as well. Once all the target groups and messages have been identified, the most credible senders and the most appropriate communication channels need to be located for each group.

There is often great disparity in the credibility of senders from group to group, and these need to be selected with a great deal of care. Credibility involves perception of expertise and trustworthiness. Effective educators must know what they are talking about and must be trusted to present it without bias. Generally, senders need to be credible with the target group before the message is sent or the message is likely to be ignored.

The communication channel is likewise important, and again, messages should be fed into channels already used by the target group whenever possible. If for example, a community program for mothers of young children is being prepared, mid-morning radio spots spoken by the President of the Parent Teachers Association might be an effective way of reaching them.

It has been established that low income families benefit from face-to-face communication more than from mass media. For individuals of lower socio-economic status, telephone contacts or other personal invitations would be more likely to succeed.

Such basic planning of communication is important to health educators. It is appropriate for those health educators trying to reach people outside the hospital, but is equally applicable to those doing staff development work or patient education. In each case, it's important to consider (1) the individuals who comprise the target group, (2) what messages they need, (3) what senders of information they believe, and (4) what channels they use to receive messages.

Most of the communication health educators provide will be of an informal variety, that is, it will not involve the health educator being televised or in other ways communicating formally. Indeed, the informal aspects of most communication is thought to be a major reason why hospital health education is so effective. The health educator can usually work with an individual or a small group of clients in an informal setting and engage in an educational encounter. Accordingly, principles of informal communication must be emphasized. Ten of these have been summarized in the self-rating scale shown in Exhibit 13–1.

MOTIVATION

Motives refer to those factors that stimulate action. The term usually refers to those drives and incentives that initiate the kinds of behavior that fulfill basic needs.

Educators often talk about motivation, and despair at their inability to motivate learners. As discussed in the previous chapter, the problem is often rooted in inappropriate selection of learning goals. If clients are learning what they want to or need to learn, in a manner and at a time when they are willing to learn, there obviously will not be a motivation problem. Educators who are having problems motivating learners would, therefore, do well to begin with a needs assessment and ascertain what the client needs or wants.

It is also appropriate to begin with client interests and to provide educational experiences that will produce results that are easily seen. Good feelings about early learning experiences are a powerful motivator for subsequent participation in educational settings.

There are also behaviors of educators that are conducive to client motivation. A dozen of these are summarized briefly below:

1. Inspire confidence of clients. It is important to act professionally and to model good behavior, though professional behavior may alienate some clients. Establish a business-like atmosphere, yet one that is warm and accepting.
   The positive effect of role models is now being documented in research, but it has been known for years that a good example adds credence to good teaching. Maintaining an appropriate weight, not smoking, and adequately handling stress are three visible areas that may impact on teaching effectiveness of health education. That modeling effect is obviously one of the major reasons for a staff health education program, as discussed throughout this book.
2. Treat each client as an individual. It is especially important to avoid stereotypes and to establish rapport with each client. Few things are

Exhibit 13–1 Informal Communication Skills

Self-Rating Scale OK	Needs Work	
____	________	1. *Know yourself and your material.* Be prepared! Recognize your own hang-ups and limitations. Express self-confidence through voice, eye contact, mannerisms, etc.
____	________	2. *Know your target group.* Learn their names and as much about their needs and interests as you can.
____	________	3. *Establish a setting conducive to communication.* Some degree of comfort and privacy is important, as is freedom from distractions.
____	________	4. *Establish rapport.* Introduce yourself. Help the respondent to feel comfortable and at ease. What happens in the first few minutes is crucial to the success of the rest of the encounter. Act interested!
____	________	5. *Clarify the problem.* Be sure you are talking about the same thing. Use probing skills often but gently.
____	________	6. *Listen actively.* Hearing is a physical process. Listening is a mental/emotional process that involves meaning.
____	________	7. *Paraphrase and reassure.* Paraphrasing helps the client to hear what he/she has said. It is also a check on your listening skills.
____	________	8. *Watch for nonverbal clues.* Meaning can be assessed by tone, loudness, pace, distance, bodily tension, posture, eye gaze, etc. Be alert to what you are communicating nonverbally.
____	________	9. *Pace your discussion.* People learn at different rates. Going too slow or fast inhibits communications.
____	________	10. *Provide feed-back.* Clearly state the conclusions reached. Probe for understanding. Work for acceptance and commitment. Leave the opportunity for additional discussion at a later time.

a more powerful persuader than a genuine interest in a client. Try to establish a helping, supporting relationship, rather than an adversary relationship. People tend to feel more cooperative if they feel accepted and not judged.

3. Try to establish a connection between the wants and needs of a client and the recommended course of action. It is always important to establish the relevance of the recommended behavior to the client.
4. Work with the client and try to identify incentives that might be effective for that client. Intrinsic motivations, such as, feelings of achievement and self-satisfaction, are worth focusing on and are usually preferable to extrinsic motivators. However, extrinsic motivators, that is, rewards of various kinds, can be effectively worked into the educational process. The behavior modification approach emphasizes such incentives.
5. Establish client goals realistically, both in short-range and long-range terms. Be sure that the task is divided into meaningful parts that will not overwhelm the client. The objectives must be as clear as possible so that the client will know exactly what has to be done, and in what sequence.
6. Work toward getting the clients to "own" their goals or plans so that behavior change is something they want to do rather than something staff wants them to do. It is appropriate to "seed ideas," including, but not limited to, attributing ideas to the client. It is especially important to work toward a verbal contract, some sense of commitment that the client will attempt to implement the behavior change.
7. Involve people in the rationale for behavior change and in the discussion of alternatives in the decision-making process when possible. Think out loud with the client. Those who are given reasons for the change are most likely to accept the change. The fullest compliance with a new procedure usually results from the fullest understanding of it.
8. Organize and present new information in a way that makes sense to the client. Relate new tasks to what is already known. Always augment ideas discussed with written instructions. Also be sure that all questions are answered, and encourage further contact if questions remain.
9. Minimize high anxiety levels and downplay failure. Maximize feelings of self-worth whenever possible. People tend to resist changes that are perceived as lowering their status. They tend to accept change that is perceived as increasing their status. Success is more

motivating than failure. Mild anxiety may be motivating, but fear may inhibit an appropriate response or may even precipitate an antagonistic response.

10. When someone objects or is in other ways negative, let them verbalize their negative response. Let them "blow off steam" but you must "maintain your cool." Establish that you understand what the client is feeling and why. Very often the client will realize that their own initial objection needs to be revised and much of the resistance will then dissipate.
11. Stimulate a sense of readiness to act that includes an understanding of the need for behavior change. Work toward a sense of immediacy. Feelings of remoteness interfere with action. Work toward the client having a sense of a "felt need" for the behavior change.
12. Reinforce good behavior whenever possible. Recognize and praise even the smallest positive response. Likewise, review and reinforce discussions and good intentions when the opportunity presents itself.

CONCLUSION

People are motivated to support ideas and concepts that agree with their basic values and to attack ideas that are opposed to their values. The more health educators can be sensitive to the individual uniqueness of each person, the more effective their efforts will be in changing the behavior of others.

An important element in health education is to be certain there is communication with the individual or group. People have minds of their own, and it is their perceptions that make them decide to act or not act. The more sensitive educators are to a particular person at a particular place and time, the more they can tie their communications into the values structure of that client. The key to good health education is to think in terms of the perspective of the client rather than the more traditional perspective of the health care providers.

REFERENCES

Mico, Paul R. and Ross, Helen S. *Health Education and Behavioral Sciences.* Oakland, Ca.: Third Party Associates, 1975.

Redman, Barbara Klug. *The Process of Patient Teaching in Nursing.* 4th rev. ed. St. Louis: C. V. Mosby Company, 1980. (Chapter 3.)

Chapter 14

Assessing Client Needs, Interests, and Learnings

14

INTRODUCTION

Health educators are constantly called upon to make learning assessments. Such judgments are made at the beginning and end of the learning process, but should also be done at all intervening stages. Assessments are often done intuitively and are more accurate if the staff member doing the assessment knows the client well. However, there are techniques which can standardize and improve the process of making these judgments. Such techniques are the focus of this chapter.

ASSESSMENT OF CLIENT NEEDS AND INTERESTS

As has been noted elsewhere in this book, effective health education needs to be individualized as much as possible. In doing so, relevance to personal needs and interests should be the major factor involved in the selection of content, methods, and materials.

The basic technique for assessing a client's needs and interests is in an intake interview. The intake interview ought to assess the client's physical and emotional needs, and other factors that impinge on educational needs. A sample intake interview form is illustrated in Exhibit 14–1.

If the client is an inpatient, it is appropriate and usually useful to monitor the patient's chart to determine diagnosis and prognosis. This permits much more focused discussion during the interview. The diagnosis and stage of the illness often provides direct input to the determination of what education is needed. Differing content or at least differing emphasis is usually needed for those in advanced stages, as opposed to those in early stages of an illness. Prognosis is of obvious importance in suggesting learning needs that will prepare the patient for that anticipated condition.

Physical Readiness

Physical readiness also includes a consideration of the levels of pain, fatigue, and other factors that affect the level of comfort. Maslow's "Hierarchy of Needs"[1] suggests that physical needs take priority over learning needs. If the patient is simply too ill to learn, then the timing is not right for the educational process. Patient readiness is critical to effective learning and teaching.

An assessment of the physical needs of a patient will also include identification of any impairments that might impede or modify the learning process. Visual, hearing, speech, or mental impairments ought to be noted and considered when assessing the client's educational needs.

Emotional Readiness

Emotional readiness to learn is based on many factors, one of which is previous educational experience in formal schooling. Negative experiences in such schooling may carry over into a hospital health education program. Another factor relates to in what stage in the acceptance process the patient is in reference to the intake diagnosis. It has been established that most patients go through several stages of acceptance, similar to those of death and dying postulated by Elisabeth Kubler Ross.[2]

This emotional readiness is also based in part on the rapport that is established between the client and the educational staff. It is also influenced by the level of support given to the educational program by physicians and other hospital staff, as perceived by the patient. There is more likely to be interest and willingness to participate if the patient is getting uniform messages that the program is important instead of the mixed signals that all too often occur. Similarly, programs aimed at staff need to have strong administrative support. Efforts expended in getting such support are usually well worthwhile.

Emotional readiness is also influenced in great measure by members of the family and significant others. They often need to be brought into both the assessment and educational process. A full assessment of the client's learning needs can on occasion not be made until the educational staff has had direct contact with close relatives and friends.

This contact with relatives and friends should also focus on any unique situations in that family's home. Any culturally-based factors need to be identified and financial factors need to be discussed openly as well. Problems with transportation, child care, and work schedules of adults in the family all may have a bearing and should be explored to determine what that impact might be.

A client's educational needs will also vary with habits and other components of life style. Smoking and drinking habits, exercise patterns, eating habits, stress reduction activities, and use of preventive measures like breast self-examination, physical exams, blood pressure monitoring, etc. can be of importance. Such a summary of life style factors is often incorporated into the health history and may be available there. If not, it should be taken as part of an educational needs assessment.

Evaluation Process

Educators need to be constantly careful not to leap to conclusions based on stereotypes or first impressions. The importance of a discussion or discussions where staff and clients get to know each other, and in which such perceptions are checked out cannot be overstressed. It is also important that whenever possible, the needs assessment should be done in a multidisciplinary manner. Patient care conferences are useful in this respect. The shared and integrated perceptions of a patient's needs will usually be more accurate than that of an individual staff member.

Entry level knowledge about the disease or disorder should be assessed. Again, this can be done informally in a discussion or an interview. Having educational protocol well-developed can assist staff in determining what concepts are understood, what concepts need to be clarified and reinforced, and what concepts need to be taught as new material.

If the evaluation process calls for measuring the attainment of knowledge or the changing of attitudes, scales will have to be developed to be administered on a pretest as well as a posttest basis. Pretesting should usually be done in the first or second session with the client.

When involved with staff or community health education programs, questionnaires are most often used to determine client needs and interests. A brief questionnaire can be used to gather the same kinds of data discussed in the previous paragraphs. The questionnaire can be required as part of the enrollment process, done before the program begins, or at the first session. It is important to get first hand information about the clients who will actually be enrolled as learners, if the learning experience is to be tailored to their needs and interests.

Exhibit 14–1 Health Education Intake Interview

Name ______________________ Chart # __________

Address ______________________________________

______________________ Telephone ____________

Referring physician ____________________________

Health education program _______________________

Age ______ Sex ______ Primary language used __________

Educational level _______________________________

Living arrangements _____________________________

Close relatives or friends _________________________

Physical readiness to learn _______________________

Emotional readiness to learn ______________________

Previous experience with the disease ________________

____

Current knowledge about the disease ________________

____

Relevant life style factors needing attention ___________

____

Preferred method(s) of learning ____________________

____

____

Intake interviewer ______________

Date ______________

Educational plan:

Signed: ________________ Date ______________

ASSESSMENT OF CLIENT LEARNINGS

It is not safe to assume that a topic that has been taught has been learned. It is necessary to constantly assess what has been learned and to review and reinforce that learning whenever possible. It is likewise useful to base teaching on existing knowledge. Both those who would teach and those who would learn need to have some sense of the beginning point, the present knowledge level, and the desired learning goal. While staff often do this routinely, the results of such assessment is often not formalized sufficiently so that it can be communicated to clients or other staff. Likewise, the more formal measurement devices are often required of programs that receive outside funds.

Observation Techniques

When assessing client progress, impressions and observations are useful though generally insufficient techniques. An assessment of a client's ability to perform a skill is best done by observing the skill being performed. Yet even this may be formalized and thus become more useful. While a relatively simple skill like administration of insulin by injection can be observed as an entity, more complex skills like use of respiratory therapy equipment or the use of biofeedback equipment may well require the use of checklists. The checklists can also be useful in the instructional phase by reminding learners of preparatory steps, of the phases or steps in the actual procedures, and those indexes of effective performance of the skill itself. Such checklists are relatively easy to prepare, but may be already available, as for example in teaching cardiopulmonary resuscitation, or in the operation of in-home inhalation therapy equipment.

Another indication of the level of patient learning is the patient's ability to verbalize what has been learned. Admittedly, the ability to verbalize is a measure of short-term understanding, and doesn't guarantee utilization. But if a patient is unable to verbalize what has been taught, there is little likeliood that the information is understood well enough to be applied. Again, this can be checked out somewhat informally in patient contacts. In these conversations, ascertain if the patient understands what is to be done. If a patient is able to discuss the procedure intelligently, at least short-term comprehension can be assumed. As was noted in the chapter on record keeping, such comprehension should be entered into the records via signed anecdotal notes. A record of what was taught and the staff's perception of the level of comprehension can be an important factor in liability suits.

When assessing client learnings, it is important to observe nonverbal factors while the patient is verbalizing what has been comprehended. Facial expressions can provide clues to the level of competency, as can the quickness and ease of the response, the tone of voice, etc. As with most communication, often how it is said will convey more of a message than what is said. Admittedly, such subjective analysis is prone to errors of interpretation. However, if the assessments are done on more than one occasion by more than one staff member, the assessments can be accurate enough to be useful. Multiple measures are basic to most learning assessment programs.

Formal Measures

Again, as noted earlier, if changes in knowledge and attitudes are being measured, more formal pretests and posttests are required. Such a procedure is more time-consuming to prepare and administer and requires a considerable amount of skill and practice to prepare effectively. Those who desire to construct such measuring devices would be well-advised to consult the many books on the topic, or better yet, seek expert assistance from those with experience in their use.

It is also consistent with the andragogical approach to health education to build in self-evaluation procedures. Learners should be encouraged to write down questions whenever they occur and ask them at an appropriate time. Brief quizzes can be given for self-evaluation with references to material covered in each question. The learning objectives can be identified in detail and made available to the group of learners so that both the clients and staff will know where they are and where they are going.

CONCLUSION

The true test of whether learning has occurred is if it is applied. Cognitive information may be obtained, and attitudes may be affected positively in the affective domain. But if behavior change does not result with the passage of time, most education has not achieved its goal. If action decisions are not impacted, little has been accomplished. As discussed in Chapter 11, follow-up measures several months after discharge are perhaps the best measure of learning and program impact. While they are time-consuming and often expensive to do, they are worth the effort periodically on at least a sample of patients.

NOTES

1. A. H. Maslow, *Motivation and Personality* (New York: Harper and Row, Publishers, 1954).
2. Elisabeth Kubler-Ross, *On Death and Dying* (New York: MacMillan Co., 1969), p. 289.

Chapter 15

Special Considerations for Special Populations

15

INTRODUCTION

Educational programs are more likely to succeed if they are tailored to the specific needs and interests of the targeted groups. While it is true that "people are people," there are three special populations that hospital health educators often work with that need special consideration: the elderly, children, and members of racial, ethnic, or class minority groups. This chapter will discuss approaches to working with each of these groups.

GERIATRIC PROGRAMS

The concept of life-long learning is one that is readily given lip service, but all too often is not emphasized in programming. Educators often accept and act out the stereotypes that the elderly can't learn very well, if at all. All elderly persons often get labeled as senile, slow, forgetful, disinterested in the real world, and living in the past. Senility is, of course, a disease process that does occur in some elderly patients, but many nonsenile patients are labeled and treated as senile, albeit unjustly.

Common sense should dispel the idea that the elderly can't learn, since millions of older adults are learning every imagined subject in formal adult education programs.[1] A study of nursing home patients with an average age of 84, found them involved in high school completion courses, college courses, current events activities, and other such programs.[2]

It is true that the aged as a group perform more poorly than young people on learning tests. However, it has been established that this poorer performance on tests is often due to noncognitive reasons, such as, poor motivation, lack of confidence, or poor conditions for learning. In other words, older people can often learn as well as younger persons, but for noncognitive reasons, are unable or unwilling to demonstrate what they have learned.

It has been established that older people learn more slowly. There is a slight decline in various mental abilities, but this decline is not usually of the magnitude to have much practical significance, other than that they may need more time than is usually allowed for learning. The concept of self-paced learning seems especially critical for the aged.

The relevance of the material is also critical, in that it affects motivation. When the relevance of the information is apparent, the older learner is often the better learner. They usually have more and better organized experiences which provide a meaningful context into which new information can be assimilated. They know themselves better and can more clearly perceive what new items of learning will be most useful to them.[3]

Care should be taken when educating the elderly to assess and meet their mental and emotional needs. As a group, the elderly are more susceptible to loneliness and depression than other groups, especially if they live alone. When they are not feeling well, it becomes easy for them to believe the stereotypes about the elderly. It is also easy for them to become intimidated by the hospital environment and to withdraw within themselves.

The elderly often need to simply be with people and reenter normal social activities. Again, staff should beware of stereotypes, in as much as many elderly people are very social and extremely busy people. Patients who appear withdrawn or reluctant to participate in educational activities should be encouraged and supported to participate in routine hospital activities instead of being forced to do so. Group learning activities are a useful way of meeting socialization and learning needs at once.

The elderly should be treated with the same respect and dignity accorded to any other human being. Educators need to treat them as individuals and work to forget the stereotypes. It is also important not to overreact and patronize elderly persons. They should be called by name, rather than "gramma."

A major concern for many elderly persons is the loss of independence, so it is important to their emotional well-being for staff not to be overly helpful. They should be allowed and encouraged to do as much as possible for themselves. It is also well to remember not to overreact to problems that occur. Small things often become increasingly important to the elderly, and if staff members are mildly distressed, it may become a major source of distress for the elderly patient.

Also important to the elderly patient's sense of well-being is that lost roles be replaced with new activities so that a major gap is not created. Staff need to be alert to what roles patients can no longer do and strive to assist the patient to either find new ways to do it or find a replacement activity for the lost role.

Health education programs for the elderly also need to be very practical. The practical matter of cooking for one, getting exercise in a shopping mall during bad weather, and keeping track of medications are all items that can be stressed.

Elderly patients often have hearing and vision problems that need to be compensated for, with communication problems the result. Again as noted in an earlier chapter, if communication doesn't occur, education does not occur. Educators have to be certain that they are effectively communicating, even though hearing and vision problems exist.

For clients who have hearing problems, it is important to speak directly to them. Some elderly patients have developed the ability to compensate by reading lips, and facial expressions help all people to comprehend more quickly. It should also be remembered to speak slowly and in lower tones. Loss of ability to hear higher tones is common in the elderly. It is usually not necessary to shout, and this is distracting to an elderly person. Speaking in normal ways is recommended, but with close attention to nonverbal feed-back to ascertain if instruction is being heard, so that the volume can be adjusted as necessary. Sentences should be short and simple with abstractions avoided.

Vision deficiency may also be a problem, though vision problems can often be more readily corrected than hearing ones. None the less, it is important to determine that the patient or patients can see adequately. They need a direct line of vision and need to be close enough to see properly any time visual aids are used. If chalkboards or posters are being used, it is important to use big print with bright colors on a light background.

In general, it is important not to underestimate or overestimate the abilities of the elderly. If needs, interests, and abilities are properly assessed, good teaching and learning can occur that will be enormously satisfying to both the patient and the educator.

There are many excellent opportunities for hospital health educators to work with the elderly in the community, as well as with those who are inpatients. Senior citizen housing complexes exist in most areas. Those staffing such programs are usually most receptive to educational activities presented by hospital staff. Ample opportunity exists to program for nutrition, exercise, medications, emotional needs, emergency medical care, and other self-help activities.

PEDIATRIC PROGRAMS

Most health educators realize that attitudes, values, and many health habits are established in the childhood years. Similarly, most health educators decry the lack of good health education in the schools. Yet many of these same health educators are not utilizing the opportunities that are available to them in their practices. So it is with hospital health educators. If, indeed, children's experiences form the basis of their attitudes toward the hospital throughout adulthood, every effort should be made to insure that that experience is a good one. Indeed, the hospital experience can be turned into an educational experience.

Ability to learn should not be a factor in the majority of children. It has been established that children have developed 80 percent of their intellectual potential by age eight.[4] As in programs for other populations, material presented will have to be relevant to their needs and interests, but assuming that as a given, children can learn about their health while hospitalized. Indeed, given the literature on "teachable moments," it may be the very best time and place to learn about health.

It is also a given that pediatric programs must include parent education. Parents need to know how to care for their child when released, but also need to know what the child has learned in order to reinforce that learning. Material for the child to take home is one good way to enhance parent and child dialogue that will result in learning for both.

Educational methods and material used is certainly another way in which a pediatric program will be unique. Activity books, games, simulations, short discussions, frequent reviews of media presentations, puppets, songs, plays, visits to other units in the hospital, and visits from staff of other units are all important ways to enhance learning among hospitalized children.

There is also an excellent opportunity to work with the elementary or nursery schools or youth groups in the community. Tours, field trips, and simple demonstrations with x-rays can be important foundations on which teachers, parents, and others can build.

In general, if pediatric educational experiences involve personal experience, hands-on activities, appropriate media, and the parents, children will learn what they need and want to learn and will enjoy doing it.

MINORITY GROUPS*

Program planners usually address programs being developed to the majority of the constituents they anticipate serving, and appropriately so.

*Hugh Blanding, M.P.H., Ph.D., community organization and urban health specialist at Central Michigan University is a major contributor to this section.

Minority groups, however, usually bring a different set of perceptions, needs, and interests with them to health education. Therefore, in order to maximize learning, it is sometimes necessary to adjust content or methodology to the individual needs and interests of clients. Perception of need frequently varies from group to group, and it is always appropriate to respond to these felt needs. Flexibility is an important quality for health educators to acquire.

Specific groups that have minority status will vary from urban to rural settings, from region to region, and from country to country. They usually consist of ethnic, racial, or class groups. Seldom do these factors operate independently of each other.[5] Health problems, attitudes toward services, and attitudes toward prevention all vary with minority status, and usually are interpreted negatively by health care providers.[6]

Characteristics of lower socio-economic Caucasians often resemble those of lower socio-economic ethnic or racial group members. Conversely, the health status and related behaviors of middle and upper class minority group members more closely resemble that of middle or upper class Caucasians. It has been determined that income and education are greater factors than race or ethnicity in determining health problems, utilization of health services, and attitudes toward educational services.[7] Staff flexibility and program adaptation are usually needed for lower socio-economic group members, regardless of racial or ethnic characteristics.

However, lower socio-economic group members who are also part of an ethnic or racial minority are more likely to be suspicious of and reticent to participate in a health education program, generally while finding such offerings unacceptable. Such responses are based partly on real or perceived lack of program relevance, and partly on conflict with enculturated values, such as, reliance on family members with folk remedies and suspicion of "white" medicine. "Distrust, fear, anger and ill will are not uncommon."[8] Such attitudes also have some of their origins in past experience and in ethnic or racial pride. It is often accentuated by lessened accessibility to health care and preventive services and lower than average health status.

The lack of knowledge and understanding often combine to create a fatalistic attitude more likely to exist in minority groups, resulting in less likelihood of follow-through on programs or in inconsistent behavior. Medical sociologists have explored this topic in much detail and have produced a great deal of literature on the topic. This brief introduction to ethnic, racial, and class differences, however, suggests that special attention should be given to members of these minority groups when they participate in health education programs.

Some beginning words of caution are in order. The advice is not new, but has not yet been widely implemented. Educators need to be ever alert that their own feelings and behaviors are not based on distortions, stereotypes, or prejudices. They also need to be alert for any stereotypes and prejudices that members of minority groups bring with them to the educational encounter.

As has been stressed throughout this book, it is imperative that health educators know their clientele as much as possible, and that programs become individualized as much as possible so that needs and interests are met. Few people consciously act on stereotypes or prejudices, though many continue to do so unaware that such feelings interfere with the educational process.

It is helpful, though not essential, when some of the educational staff are members of the minority group being served. It will probably be true that hospitals serving large Oriental, Chicano, American Indian, or Black populations will have members of these groups on their staff in some capacity. Programs can often be enhanced by such personnel, making it easier to establish rapport and communication.

Communication can be a critical problem, ranging from the problems of a refugee who can't speak English to Americans who have dialects or idioms that are different from those of the staff. Some programs have experimented with employing health aides from the minority groups being served, training them to do a specific program. Some problems are circumvented with such programming, while others may be created. Whatever approach is used, it must be remembered that communication must occur before education can be effective.

Health educators need to constantly remember that the "human touch" can and does often transcend any cultural or class differences that may exist between clients and staff. The ability of staff to empathize becomes critical. Sincerity of purpose must be manifested in nonverbal ways. Staff "openness" increases in importance, if trust is to develop. More personal contact, personal interest in the "whole" person, dialogue, and support often are helpful.

Clients should not be inundated with attention just because they are members of a minority group. While it is improbable that staff can care too much, it is possible that staff can do so much for a client that it is interpreted by the client as being demeaning.

Another major area of concern is in the area of educational materials. Materials should in so far as is possible be relevant to the real world of the patient. It is often difficult for the rural poor to grasp the significance of a teaching film placed in the setting of a large metropolitan area. Dietary adjustments and other aspects of home health care must be placed in the real parameters of a patient's world in order to maximize learning. Home visitations are one way to enhance this if staffing permits. Unfortunately, it often does not.

It should be noted that minority group members have many of the same learning needs as others. Generally speaking, commonalities should be accented and differences should be minimized. Minorities may have difficulty seeing the relevance or feasibility of applying the learning to their particular life setting. Staff need to be more concerned that the relevance is clear to the learner when the learner's frame of reference is different from their own. Staff should also be certain that their interest and concern in each patient is genuine and is expressed in both verbal and nonverbal manners.

CONCLUSION

The basic principles of health education include doing a needs assessment, establishing rapport and communication, and individualizing the instruction so as to meet identified needs. Relevance to reality is also always important but is especially crucial to special populations.

All the basic principles apply to efforts in programming for special populations, but some additional considerations as suggested in this chapter may have to be made to maximize potential learning. Those who have been involved in such efforts have found that it works, and that it can be extremely rewarding. Special considerations for special populations can pay big dividends to the health education program.

NOTES

1. Roger DeCrow, *New Learning for Older Americans* (Washington, D.C.: Adult Education Association of the U.S.A., 1974), p. 2.
2. Donald J. Breckon, "Patient Education Programs in Michigan Nursing Care Facilities" (Ph.D. diss., Michigan State University, 1977).
3. Diana Woodruff and David Walsh, "Research in Adult Learning," *The Gerontologist* 15 (1975): 425.
4. Anne Impellizzeri and Lynne Bernstein, *Health Education of Preschool Children and Their Parents* (Lansing Mi.: Society for Public Health Education, Great Lakes Chapter, 1975), p. 5.
5. Thomas Pettigrew, "Race and Class in the 1980's: An Interactive View," *Daedalus* 2 (1981): 233.
6. *Health Status of Minorities and Low Income Groups* (Washington, D.C.: U.S. Department of Health, Education, and Welfare, 1979), p. 11.
7. Ibid., p. 207.
8. Paul Adams, "Black Patients and White Doctors," *Urban Health* 6, no. 6 (1977): 22.

REFERENCE

Daedalus, Journal of American Academy of Arts and Sciences, "American Indians, Blacks, Chicanos, and Puerto Ricans," Spring 1981.

Chapter 16

Ethics for Hospital Health Educators*

*Adapted from Donald J. Breckon and Karen Ledebuhr, "Ethics for Patient Education," from *Health Values*, May 1981 by permission of Charles Slack Inc., Thorofare, N.J.

16

INTRODUCTION

Ethics are variously defined as a "set of moral principles or values," "principles of conduct governing an individual or group," or "the discipline of dealing with what is good and bad."[1] It translates into what are acceptable standards of conduct for members of a profession.

The AMA states in the preamble to its Principles of Medical Ethics that ethics "are not laws but standards by which a physician may determine the propriety of his conduct in his relationship with patients, with colleagues, with members of the allied professions, and with the public."[2] It seems apparent that all professional groups ought to have clearly defined and widely publicized ethical standards.

EVOLUTION OF ETHICAL STANDARDS IN HEALTH CARE

Ethical standards usually evolve as a discipline matures. They grow out of a myriad of experiences in which behavior is discussed and judged as appropriate or inappropriate. They grow out of a discussion of the "rightness" of behavior in specific situations, and related questions, such as, "what should I have done?" or "what would you have done?" The answers to such questions and the results of such discussions are then generalized and codified, usually by a committee. They are developed into a system of guidelines that will assist the practicing professional in making moral decisions in future situations of difficulty faced on the job.

The ethical standards that evolve must be situational in nature. Accordingly, licensure boards cannot test for compliance in advance. But standards that have been developed can be taught to those preparing to enter the profession. Case studies can be used to explore when individual standards might be applicable.

Ethical statements can also be used in court cases. If a practicing professional can demonstrate that he or she complied with those ethical standards developed and approved by peers, the likelihood of a negative judgment being rendered will be reduced.

As noted above, the AMA has officially adopted Principles of Medical Ethics. So has the American Nurses' Association (ANA)[3] and the Society for Public Health Education (SOPHE).[4] Patient education is a rapidly emerging discipline that cuts across the three fields cited above and has been endorsed and/or mandated at the state and federal level by several regulating or funding agencies. Students are being trained for patient education positions and are being awarded degrees in that specialty. Job descriptions have been written, and many specialists are currently practicing in the field. Newsletters, journals, books, and other materials have been and continue to be prepared for their use. It is apparent that the time has arrived to develop a system of ethics that apply specifically to this emerging discipline of patient education.

ETHICAL ISSUES

In examining the ethical codes of the three professional organizations mentioned above, the AMA, the ANA, and the SOPHE, it becomes evident that there are four major areas of concern covered: (1) relationships with individual patients; (2) responsibility for the public welfare; (3) obligations to colleagues and self, and (4) relationships with other health care professionals. These statements address common issues, sometimes differing only in wording, while at times addressing the unique aspects of each profession. An examination of these issues provides insights to patient educators.

Relationships With Individual Patients

Two primary issues are addressed in all three codes. First, the professional must respect the dignity of the patient. Second, the professional must respect the individual's right to privacy and must maintain confidentiality.

The ANA and SOPHE codes suggest that the professional must respect the uniqueness and worth of the individual and must not discriminate concerning whom they will serve. The AMA code, in contrast, suggests the physician "may choose whom he will serve,"[5] except in the case of an emergency.

The Professional's Responsibility for the Public Welfare

Two issues involving responsibility for public welfare are discussed in all three ethical codes reviewed. The professional is obligated to be concerned with and active in assisting the public to meet its health needs. However, each of the codes suggest a different method for promoting the health of the public. The AMA suggests "participation in activities which have the purpose of improving both the health and well being of the individual and the community."[6] The AMA recognizes the possibilities of a conflict between an individual's welfare and the public good, but does not offer definitive guidelines for dealing with the conflict.

The ANA code suggests that "the nurse participates in the profession's efforts to protect the public from misinformation and misrepresentation."[7] The ANA code further requires that the nurse participate in a team approach to meet the public's health needs. SOPHE's code suggests yet another emphasis, "Health educators will aid the consumer public in making informed judgments and choices on matters that concern them."[8]

Professionals are, in general, urged to assist in protecting the public against unprofessional practices, variously described as unethical, incompetent, or illegal in nature. All three codes are quite specific in requiring the professional to be alert for other professionals whose practices are suspect and to take action against such people. The AMA limits such actions to the policing of its own members, while the ANA holds the nurse responsible for taking action against any health care professional.

Professional Obligations to Colleagues and Self

The three codes reviewed all stated that the professional is obligated to maintain and improve his or her capabilities on a continuing basis so as to be of maximum benefit to those served. The professional is also charged with furthering the growth and development of the profession through participation in research and philosophical discussions, and to share the results of such investigations with professional colleagues.

Professionals are also urged to develop and maintain a professional environment. The reference is to an environment that will not interfere with or impair delivering of quality care,[9] and free exercise of judgment,[10] and nurturing the individual's growth and development.[11]

Relationships with Other Health Care Professionals

Professionals are urged to work within the boundaries of standard accepted practices associated with the profession and to use consultants or refer to other more specialized colleagues when appropriate. The AMA urges members not to receive a commission for referrals and supports the use of consultations to enhance quality care. The ANA code speaks to the issue of delegating activities to others who may not be competent, yet emphasizes a good working relationship with the health care team. The SOPHE code requires that the health educator make his or her intentions known to others who are involved in a case, especially when conflicts arise.

A BEGINNING POINT

The review of issues covered in the three codes makes it obvious that there are some issues of common concern to all who work in the health care field. Likewise, there are some statements that deal with unique aspects of a profession. These two observations suggest that any ethical code for patient education ought to include the basics common to all professions, but ought to also be specific to the situations that that group of professionals is likely to confront. It also suggests that there is a need for a statement of ethics that is specific to each group of health care professionals.

The following 16 statements, then, are proposed as a basis for more conversation that will hopefully lead to the adoption of a code of ethics specifically for hospital health educators. The hospital health educator:

1. Practices nondiscrimination and provides educational services to whomever needs them, regardless of age, sex, race, handicap, or state of health.
2. Respects the dignity and worth of each client, recognizing his or her uniqueness and treats the client as an individual.
3. Recognizes and respects prevalent beliefs, values, and practices of community groups and subgroups.
4. Grants each client privacy and confidentiality, unless released from this assumed commitment by the client. The health educator is especially careful about casual conversations about a client in front of other clients, family, or friends.
5. Recognizes and works constructively with family members or other people identified by the client to be significant to his or her health care. The health educator endeavors to strengthen ties to others that will benefit the client.
6. Supports the principle of informed consent and extends it to participation in health education programs.
7. Makes clear the purposes, commitments, responsibilities, and limitations of the professional relationship with clients in educational

programs. The health educator endorses the concept of the client accepting responsibility for his or her health and works to achieve that goal.

8. Prefers and strives to achieve active participation of the patient in both the learning process and in the planning and evaluation of that learning. The health educator endorses the goal of life-long learning and helps the patient find meaning, satisfaction, and self-fulfillment in learning.
9. Recognizes and compensates for physical defects of clients, such as vision and hearing problems, language barriers, etc.
10. Recognizes and addresses the problems of emotional stress associated with the early stages of many illnesses.
11. Participates in professional continuing education on a regular basis, endeavoring to keep up with the state of the art. The health educator attends conferences and annual meetings and keeps up with the literature of the profession.
12. Practices within the boundaries of sound health education theory, standard accepted practices, and his or her own professional expertise. The health educator accepts responsibility for such practices and beliefs.
13. Evaluates his or her professional practice continuously, and maintains an image of professional competency and decorum that is above reproach. Specifically, the health educator avoids any practices that might be interpreted by others as unethical, unprofessional, illegal, or otherwise inappropriate.
14. Is alert for and takes action to protect clients from others who practice behaviors that endanger the well-being of the client. The health educator always works through appropriate channels when initiating any such actions.
15. Continually evaluates programs and conducts research in an effort to further the body of health education knowledge and practice, and maintain the integrity of health education.
16. Uses a teamwork approach, seeking a consulting, cooperative effort that will benefit the client.

CONCLUSION

The attention of educators and administrators to ethical standards will pay dividends in the maintenance of quality and the development of confidence. All who play leadership roles should promote high standards of practice and model them. To do otherwise is shortsighted and self-defeating. A profession like education that is built on trust, voluntary participation, and voluntary compliance must, if it is to succeed, maintain standards of practice that are above reproach.

NOTES

1. *Webster's New World Dictionary of the American Language* (New York: World Publishing Co., 1972), p. 220.
2. *Principles of Medical Ethics* (Chicago: American Medical Association, 1978).
3. *Code for Nurses* (Kansas City: American Nurses' Association, 1976).
4. *Code of Ethics* (San Francisco: Society for Public Health Education, 1976).
5. AMA, *Principles of Medical Ethics.*
6. AMA, *Principles of Medical Ethics.*
7. ANA, *Code for Nurses.*
8. SOPHE, *Code of Ethics.*
9. AMA, *Principles of Medical Ethics.*
10. ANA, *Code for Nurses.*
11. SOPHE, *Code of Ethics.*

Chapter 17

The Future of Hospital Health Education*

*Reprinted from Donald J. Breckon, "Futures in Patient Education," *Michigan Hospitals* 17, no. 1 (January 1980), by permission of Michigan Hospital Association, © 1980.

17

INTRODUCTION

It is important for present and potential practitioners in the field to contemplate the future and what it holds for health education. The past and the present are largely beyond change. Educators can, however, learn from the past and present. As Alvin Toeffler suggests, if we do not, we shall be compelled to relive it, and even worse, to endure the future we have created.

The future is created with a series of choices, not always made deliberately or collectively. The choices are usually swayed by many external and internal forces. External forces often include such factors as funding, administrative support, legislation, and technology. Internal forces include such factors as commitment of time, energy, and influence which one author refers to as the "scarcities of abundance."[1] Given such commitment, hospital health educators can choose to shape the future, just as the United States government chose to put a man on the moon in eight years.

Some futurists believe anything can be accomplished in twenty years, if enough planning and commitment are present. What society chooses to do about hospital health education will, in large measure, depend on the commitment of time, energy, and influence that is made. Unfortunately, the choices are often in reality a failure to choose any course of action, which is recognized as a decision only after a prolonged time of drifting. Not to choose to shape the future is a course of action that most rational people would not choose deliberately, but is the path of least resistance followed by many. The winds of change sometimes reach hurricane force, so educators need to chart a course and shape their future.

Hospital health educators should accept responsibility for their future; it doesn't just happen. It is important to decide what kind of future is wanted and then make it happen.

THE IMMEDIATE FUTURE

The immediate future for hospital health education is most predictable. There is a ground swell of support at the federal, state, and local level. The concept has been supported by legislators, accrediting bodies, professional associations, and consumer advocates. Professionally trained health educators are available. Adequate technology is available. Administrative support at the institutional level is admittedly still the biggest variable. While there are no perfect programs yet, an adequate job is being done on a small scale in some places.

While inflation will probably continue throughout the 1980s, efforts at controlling the rising health care costs will lead to more emphasis on health education. When a society commits itself to paying the total health care costs of a nation, it will quickly discover that it is more cost-efficient to prevent disease rather than treat it or live with its after effects.

Good health education programs will increase in the 1980s. The biggest change that will be seen is that educators will be doing well what they already know how to do. There will be programs that are adequately financed, staffed, and have good facilities and equipment. There will be sound planning procedures being used with well-designed curricula. There will be a variety of educational methodologies being available, with the educational mix being determined by a needs assessment. One-to-one instruction, small group discussion, programmed material, and audio-visual aids will all be used effectively. The instruction will be reinforced by medical and nursing staff, and will include family members so that it can also be reinforced at home. Discharge planning will occur for all patients, with written confirmation, so that all patients or those caring for them will know precisely what to do. A "hot line" will also be available for patient inquiries. There will also be good programs for hospital staff and for the community. The hospital will be in reality the center of preventive medicine for the community. All such health education programs will be adequately evaluated and revised periodically. While this may sound like it is eons away, it need not be. It is a cursory description of the state of the art at present. It will become common practice in the 1980s.

ANTICIPATED INNOVATIONS IN THE 1980s

1. Information Retrieval Systems—Large computers have the capabilities of building large data banks, and the 1980s will be an "Age of Information."[2] Information overload is already being discussed and clients and staff alike will need assistance in analyzing and utilizing this information.

Information about individual clients or about all people with a specific disorder will be readily available. Staff will know more and more about what clients have done or are likely to do than ever before. Having access to such information will assist them in being more effective in educational programming.

Computers have also created on-line libraries where information is electronically stored and is analyzed and called up on demand. Hospitals can have access to such systems and perhaps in time, in-home computers can call forth information from a centralized health education library.

2. Media Developments—Videocassettes are already available. They are being used in some hospitals as a poor substitute for a health education program. They can be used far more effectively as tools in a health education effort. Home videotape recorders now on the market will be found in one-third of the American homes by 1985 predict Wall Street analysts.[3] They will project their programs on a wall-sized screen. Cassettes prepared by health education specialists will be available and can likewise be viewed and reviewed by clients and their family.

Also expected to be popular and to have a profound effect on hospital health education are the newly introduced videodiscs.[4] Videodiscs resemble a phonograph record, but are read with laser beams. One disc is currently capable of recording 54,000 pages. They are capable of storing motion pictures, slides, or printed material. An entire set of encyclopedias could be stored on one disc. They will become cost-efficient with expanded use. Learners can be sent home with a complete health education program, carefully indexed so that the client and his or her family can play or replay the most relevant parts. Such systems will be replete with slow motion and stop action to further enhance learning. Videodiscs can fulfill the educational expectation raised but never achieved by TV, their chief advantage being the viewer can choose his or her own time to watch each lesson.

Two-way cable TV with videophones will also be available[5] and can have great potential for education of the patient who has returned home even earlier to reduce health care costs. Questions could be asked of hospital personnel from a bed at home. The two-way videotape will allow demonstrations or other kinds of prescriptive feed-back from the hospital ward.

The world has also entered into the era of microprocessors or minicomputers.[6] About one-fourth the size of a small fingernail, the silicon microprocessor makes a wide variety of complex operations possible, as in calculators and microwave ovens. Synthetic voice technology is being developed and some electronics experts predict that by the mid-1980s, they will be able to carry on simple conversations with their owners. Certainly, if a microwave oven can talk to a client in Spanish, French, German, or

English, a similar unit could be designed to answer the ten most common questions that a staff member trying to stop smoking will have.

The Bell System is planning such features as timed messages.[7] For example, a hospital could program a central recording machine to dial patients at a designated time and remind them to take their medicine. Think what that can do to compliance rates. Life-long learning can indeed become a reality.

THE 1980s AND BEYOND

Vance Packard in his book, *The People Shapers*,[8] described research of the 1970s and made projections of what might happen unless controls were instituted. He projects behavior surveillance by remote television, universal identifiers with computerized records of all transactions a person makes, and surgically implanted transmitters. Theoretically, health care personnel will have complete knowledge of a patient's behavior before and after the hospital stay. Health education personnel will not have to rely on personal recall for information on eating patterns, exercise habits, compliance with medication regimens, and work habits, to name some elements of patient behavior. If professional health educators are to shape their future, ways must be found to effectively utilize this data.

Packard also projects widespread use of human seedbanks, test tube babies, embryo transplants to professional surrogate human mothers, animals who will carry the human baby to term, or artificial wombs. Predetermination of the sex of children and their genetic endowment will be possible. Cloning, man-animal combinations, and artificial limbs and organs reminiscent of television's Bionic Man and Woman will be possible. Even head transplants will be feasible.

Behavior modification will be more sophisticated. The use of brainwashing techniques; subliminal stimulation; remote hypnosis using the electronic media, drugs, and chemicals; and the use of surgically implanted electrodes forebode complete behavior control and mood control if allowed to develop unchecked.

There are tremendous implications for hospital health education in each of these possible developments. Certainly if the techniques are available, ways ought to be found to use them constructively. Of equal certainty is the fact that each of these procedures will require a great deal of understanding about the particular advantages, disadvantages, and consequences of each action.

Certainly these and other developments suggest issues that will arise with which health education will have to deal:

1. Invasion of privacy—How much should health care personnel be allowed to learn about a client without self-disclosure or release?
2. Information overload—Will patients and staff alike be able to handle and effectively utilize the increased volume of information that is becoming available?
3. Manipulation of people's behavior—How much manipulation is tolerable? How much choice will be allowed? Who will choose? How much informed decision making will be allowed?
4. Dominance of technology—Is technology the best way to educate, even if it becomes the cheapest? Will tight budgets mean eliminating staff, and what will be the consequence of reducing human contact? Will those in the field find meaning in their work?
5. Ownership of knowledge—Will the profit motive interfere or assist in the development of good health education programs? Will "use" become the value of knowledge rather than ownership?
6. Inertia of the system—Will those who control the health care system allow health education to develop to the potential that it has?
7. Funding and accountability—Who will pay for the system; the client, the government? Will the client be required to pay for self-inflicted damage as a result of overindulgence in food, tobacco, alcohol, or the failure to exercise, reduce stress, or wear a seat belt?
8. Ethics—Who will make the decision about what's right? Who will control those who would control people's lives? Dare it be left to self-regulation? Can the government do it effectively? Are new structures needed?

Decisions regarding these issues should be based, at least in part, on the values suggested by Vance Packard.[9] High value should be placed on developments that promote (a) responsible self-direction, (b) individual fulfillment, (c) rearing of fine children, (d) uniqueness of personhood, (e) spontaneity, (f) independent thinking, and (g) freedom from coercion. Low value should be placed on developments that would (a) make people more predictable, (b) weaken family ties, (c) make people more irresponsible, (d) dehumanize or adulterate people, (e) make people more dependent on others, and (f) more malleable. Such principles ought also to guide behavior in 1980.

THE 21st CENTURY: WHERE WILL WE BE?

The 21st century is coming, whether we are ready for it or not. Who dares predict where we will be? The rate of change is fifty times what it used to be and is still increasing. The world has progressed through periods of gradual change, then rapid and radical change, to a period of convulsive change. Some have concluded it is the death struggle of a civilization. Others conclude it's the birth struggle of a new civilization emerging from the old. Which will it be? What will the future hold for patient education?

CONCLUSION

It has been said that there are three kinds of people: (1) those that make things happen, (2) those that watch things happen, and (3) those that wonder what happened. Health educators should be willing to make a significant investment in the future. After all is said and done, they are going to have to spend the rest of their lives there.

NOTES

1. Edward Cornish, *Planting Seeds for the Future* (Stamford, Ct.: Champion International Corp., 1979), p. 18.
2. Robert Stakenas and Roger Kaufman, *Educational Technology and Cost Reduction in Higher Education* (Tallahassee, Fla.: Florida State University, 1977), p. 149.
3. Susan Barker, "Fine Living," *Passenger*, March 1980, pp. 12–15.
4. Jack Margarrell, "The Imminent Videodisc Revolution," *Chronicle of Higher Education*, April 11, 1977, p. 5.
5. Robert Frizzle, *An Educational Model for the Future* (Houston: World Future Society, 1978), p. 19.
6. Thomas Held and Murray Kappelman, *Continuing Health Education Through Computer Technology* (Miami: Health Education Medical Conference, 1976), p. 11.
7. Andrew Korim, *Education and Work in the Future*, (Houston: Conference on Future of Work and the Community College, 1978), p. 27.
8. Vance Packard, *The People Shapers* (Boston: Little Brown and Company, 1977), Chapter 26.
9. Ibid.

Appendix A

AHA's A Patient's Bill of Rights, House of Delegates, February 6, 1973

Source: Reprinted with the permission of the American Hospital Association, © 1972.

appendix A

1. The patient has the right to considerate and respectful care.

2. The patient has the right to obtain from his physician complete current information concerning his diagnosis, treatment, and prognosis in terms the patient can be reasonably expected to understand. When it is not medically advisable to give such information to the patient, the information on the patient should be made available to an appropriate person in his behalf. He has the right to know by name the physician responsible for coordinating his care.

3. The patient has the right to receive from his physician information necessary to give informed consent prior to the start of any procedure and/or treatment. Except in emergencies, such information for informed consent, should include but not necessarily be limited to the specific consent, should include but not necessarily be limited to the specific procedure and/or treatment, the medically significant risks involved, and the probable duration of incapacitation. Where medically significant alternatives for care or treatment exist, or when the patient requests information concerning medical alternatives, the patient has the right to such information. The patient also has the right to know the name of the person responsible for the procedures and/or treatment.

4. The patient has the right to refuse treatment to the extent permitted by law, and to be informed of the medical consequences of his action.

5. The patient has the right to every consideration of his privacy concerning his own medical care program. Case discussion, consultation, examination, and treatment are confidential and should be conducted discreetly. Those not directly involved in his care must have the permission of the patient to be present.

6. The patient has the right to expect that all communications and records pertaining to his care should be treated as confidential.

7. The patient has the right to expect that within its capacity a hospital must make reasonable response to the request of a patient for services. The hospital must provide evaluation, service, and/or referral as indicated by the urgency of the case. When medically permissible a patient may be transferred to another facility only after he has received complete information and explanation concerning the needs for and alternatives to such a transfer. The institution to which the patient is to be transferred must first have accepted the patient for transfer.

8. The patient has the right to obtain information as to any relationship of his hospital to other health care and education institution insofar as his care is concerned. The patient has the right to obtain information as to the existence of any professional relationships among individuals by name, who are treating him.

9. The patient has the right to be advised if the hospital proposes to engage in or perform human experimentation affecting his care or treatment. The patient has the right to refuse to participate in such research projects.

10. The patient has the right to expect reasonable continuity of care. He has the right to know in advance what appointment times and physicians are available and where. The patient has the right to expect that the hospital will provide a mechanism whereby he is informed by his physician or a delegate of the physician of the patients continuing health care requirements following discharge.

11. The patient has the right to examine and receive an explanation of his bill regardless of source of payment.

12. The patient has the right to know what hospital rules and regulations apply to his conduct as a patient.

No catalogue of right can guarantee for the patient the kind of treatment he has a right to expect. A hospital has many functions to perform, including the prevention and treatment of disease, the education of both health professionals and patients, and the conduct of clinical research. All these activities must be conducted with an overriding concern for the patient, and, above all, the recognition of his dignity as a human being. Success in achieving this recognition assures success in the defense of the rights of the patient.

Appendix B

AMA's Statement on Patient Education, House of Delegates, June 1975

Source: Reprinted with permission of the American Medical Association, © 1975.

appendix B

Resolutions 37 and 41 (C-74) dealing with patient education were referred to the Board of Trustees for study and report at the 1975 Annual Convention.

Both resolutions called for planned programs of patient education developed and supervised by patient education committees whose membership would include health professionals, educators and consumers. Both would have required that such programs be prescribed by a physician and documented on the patient's charts, as a basis for third-party reimbursement.

The American Medical Association's Department of Health Education and Division of Medical Practice have been exploring the overall subject of planned patient education programs and have arrived at the following general findings and recommendations in response to Resolutions 37 and 41 (C-74).

DEFINITION AND ROLE OF PLANNED PATIENT EDUCATION PROGRAMS

It is recognized that increasingly complex patterns of health care, along with the patient's environment, attitude, life style and cooperation, all play an important part in effective treatment. Informed, motivated and supportive participation in treatment by patients and their families can aid the recovery of the patient and enhance the quality of his health. Patient education, as an integral part of high quality health care, provides an avenue to such improved participation.

Education of the patient has always been part of the ongoing professional responsibility of physicians, nurses, dieticians, therapists and all other members of the health team. Health professionals have traditionally provided patients with some information about their illness and the prescribed course of treatment. Some health instruction has also been provided. In some situations, there is a need indicated for a structured educational effort beyond that which individual members of the team can provide. It is in these situations that planned patient education programs may be expected to serve.

The provision of patient education services, designed to assist the patient and his family in the effective management of individual health, is a shared and continuous responsibility of both the physician and the patient. Patient education directed toward the effective management of individual illness and maintenance of health commences with the patient's entry into the health services. A positive personal experience between the physician and the patient at first contact will greatly contribute to the success of an effective patient education program.

The following factors define planned patient education:

1. Programs are distinguished from general health education of the public in that they focus on individuals who present themselves for medical services in institutions and in physicians' offices.
2. Programs are directed at the patient's understanding of his specific disease entity or physical or mental disability.
3. Programs assist the patient (and/or sometimes family members) to cooperate in the treatment of the disease or disability.
4. Programs involve patients with diseases or disabilities in which there are substantial grounds for belief that the patient will be better able to participate in treatment and that the treatment will be more effective with such a planned program than without it.

It should be clear from these four factors that planned patient education programs are distinct from general health education programs for the public and from programs intended as education for prevention of disease or for health maintenance. The planned program is for patients under treatment.

As the relationship between the physician and the patient is established, the physician determines the patient's level of knowledge concerning his illness or health, and the patient's educational needs. In this relationship, it is incumbent upon the patient to provide the necessary health history and medical information, and to comply with the prescribed medical regimen. Adherence to a prescribed treatment program is dependent upon the patient's understanding and acceptance of his condition, recognition of the importance of his role in the daily management of his prescribed treatment and satisfaction with health services provided. It is in these areas that a planned patient education program can enhance quality care.

REIMBURSEMENT

Planned patient education is a legitimate reimbursable item of patient care, when prescribed by a physician, appropriate to the patient's condition and substantiated by entries on the patient record. Planned patient education should be eligible for reimbursement under the various health insurance and other third-party payment programs.

BENEFITS

Properly planned programs of this type will improve care and can reduce the overall cost of treatment. Enabling patients to play a greater part in their own treatment can reduce unnecessary utilization of trained health professionals and of health care facilities. However, potential benefits such as cost containment, shortened recovery time and improved patient morale may not be immediately achievable. Any new interdisciplinary program takes time to develop and to become effective.

CONTENT AND ORIENTATION

Planned patient education programs should be based on identified objectives; should make use of sound educational methods; should have approved content that is scientifically accurate; and should be adaptable to the individual needs of patients.

Objectives need to be clarified at the outset along with specific criteria for measuring their achievement. The success or failure of the program should be determined by how well the objectives are realized.

RECOMMENDATIONS

The Board of Trustees believes the general findings and recommendations contained in this report respond to Resolutions 37 and 41, and recommends that the report be adopted and Association activities to improve effective patient education be continued.

Appendix C

SOPHE's Position Statement on Patient and Family Education, October 1976

appendix C

Educational programs should be planned as an integral part of high quality care and are essential to comprehensive health care delivery systems which recognize that the informed patient is an essential member of a health care team.

Irrespective of the location or situation in which care is offered, those responsible have an obligation to provide to the best of their ability an organized approach to patient education. In larger settings this will, in most instances, be a patient education committee composed of qualified health professionals representing the several multidisciplinary departments or services needed for developing sound content. This should ensure that the educational effort will be a helpful, practical process involving the use of a specific educational plan, supported by the therapeutic team, with progress notes as part of the patient's record. The practice of recording this plan is important in assessment and evaluation.

The patient should participate in establishing educational objectives that are relevant, whatever the setting: inpatient, out-patient department, community clinic, doctor's office, skilled nursing facility.

The patient and family should receive education as to the accessability of care, the system of care, and the role which each can play in prevention and treatment. The latter should include both the physical and emotional aspects of the illness.

The needs of patients and the resources available understandably set parameters within which patient education programs can be developed. The effectiveness of the education is of paramount importance and goals must therefore have specific objectives stated in measurable terms. Only then can effectiveness be evaluated.

Payment for qualified educational programs appropriate to the health needs of the patient is a legitimate part of health care costs. Since community education and preventive information programs can reduce the cost of health care, financing of such efforts should be more broadly based through joint efforts of health care facilities, organizations, foundations and governmental agencies. This involvement for financial planning should be projected for a time period of at least three years to establish a sound program and to assure continuity of services.

Qualified health educators serving as the coordinators of patient/family education programs have repeatedly demonstrated an ability to help patients change their behavior and assist the facilities and organizations they serve strengthen and broaden health services offered to consumers.

Appendix D

HIAA's Financing In-Hospital Patient Education: Proposed Criteria, 1979

Source: Reprinted from "Financing In-Hospital Patient Education: Proposed Criteria," by Health Insurance Association of America, 1979. Used with permission.

appendix D

STATEMENT OF CRITERIA

Individual responsibility plays a crucial role in solving the problems of ill health in America. The reality is that most of the causes and the treatment of illness and disability are affected by what people do to and for themselves.

It is therefore imperative that individuals achieve a better understanding of their personal health needs, and of the options and resources available to them.

Health education is the means by which illness and disability can best be prevented or its impact minimized. Basic to the health education process is its potential for encouraging more effective, efficient and economic use of health services. Especially is this true with respect to education of the hospitalized patient.

A well informed and motivated patient stands a far better chance of early recovery and is less likely to suffer a recurrence of ill health. This can lead to reduced hospital utilization rates and hence lower costs.

HOSPITAL-BASED PATIENT EDUCATION

Accordingly, the Health Insurance Association of America gives strong support to organized hospital-based patient education programs. Such programs represent one immediate opportunity for individual involvement in the medical care process.

In effect, insurance companies over the years have been reimbursing for the cost of existing patient education services included as part of a hospital's daily service charge.

Ideally, health education costs should be built into each hospital's per diem rate and borne equitably by all payors of services.

To this end, three obstacles need to be overcome:

1. The lack of incentive for physicians and hospitals to include patient education as an integral part of the treatment;
2. The lack of assurance as to whether the services are appropriate and effective;
3. The disproportionate share of hospital costs too often paid by patients out-of-pocket or under insurance company policies. This occurs when costs for patient education are identified separately and not recognized as an allowable expense item in the cost formulas of Medicare, Medicaid, and Blue Cross.

Insurance companies must serve the best interests of their policyholders. With respect to payment for patient health education, assurances are required by companies that existing programs function effectively as an integral part of the total patient care spectrum. Moreover, these costs must be reasonable and equitably shared among all purchasers of hospital services.

Certain other patient education criteria are essential, including:

1. Acceptance of standards of professional practice;
2. Approval of services and programs by the regional Health Systems Agencies established under the National Health Planning and Resources Development Act of 1974;
3. Periodic review and approval by the Joint Commission on Accreditation of Hospitals.

STANDARDS OF PRACTICE

Realistically patient education programs will vary from hospital to hospital to meet a diversity of needs. Nevertheless, there should be elements and practices common to all programs that can be defined and measured.

Model programs should be evaluated with a view toward formulating these standards of practice. The HIAA proposes that this evaluation be undertaken by the National Center for Health Education.

Acceptable standards would make it feasible for Health Systems Agencies to review the appropriateness and quality of health education and services from both the community and hospital viewpoints. Such review is particularly important for small hospitals where cooperative efforts among several institutions may be necessary—and perhaps even involving other outside agencies.

The accreditation process should have the authority to assure program accountability. If necessary, any hospital without appropriate health education procedures in place, or in development, would lose its accreditation.

Fulfillment of all of these aims calls for a total commitment withi the health education field and among the health providers, health insurers, health planning agencies, and hospital accreditation systems.

Above all, each individual in the exercise of responsibility will make the crucial difference in the management of good health. This is the expectation and goal of health education of the public as part of the broader effort to contain the costs and assure the quality of health care.

ILLUSTRATIVE CASE STUDIES ON THE COST BENEFIT OF PATIENT EDUCATION PROGRAMS

Diabetes patients participated in an educational program using as a means for obtaining information a telephone hot-line installed at a county hospital in Southern California. Over a two-year period the incidence of diabetic coma at the clinic was reduced from 300 to 100; there was a 50 percent reduction in the number of emergency room visits per diabetic patient; and approximately 2,300 medication visits were avoided. Total savings for the two years were estimated to be $1.8 million.[1]

Forty-five hemophiliac patients and their families were instructed in the selfmanagement of their condition at the Tufts-New England Medical Center. The result was a 90 percent drop in in-patient days, and 89 percent reduction in out-patient visits and a 45 percent decrease in total medical costs per patient based on pre-post comparisons.[2]

An experimental group of 26 asthmatic patients met in discussion groups at Johns Hopkins Hospital to gain a better understanding of their condition. After four months the experimental group experienced 50 percent less visits to the emergency room than the control group and it was estimated that for every dollar spent for the educational services, $6 of medical care costs were saved.[3]

One hundred congestive heart patients were assigned to experimental and control groups at a hospital in New Brunswick, New Jersey. The experimental group and their families were given a broad range of education and counseling about the disease. The experimental group patients had one-third as many readmission days, one-half the number of readmissions, and adhered more faithfully to the medical regimen.[4]

Forty-seven health educated patients with pre-operation instruction who underwent abdominal surgery at Massachusetts General Hospital went home, on the average, 2.7 days earlier than 51 patients in the control group who were given minimal information and guidance.[5]

CONCLUSION

The Health Insurance Association of America believes that health education is an essential and integral component of the total process of delivering high quality medical care, and in the development of healthful living. Health education should be designed to fulfill the following purposes:

1. Improve the quality of life of the individual, family, and the community through programs which:

    - help people understand themselves, their bodies, and their bodily systems;
    - facilitate ways by which individuals and families can protect, improve, and maintain their own health; and
    - provide useful information about illness, diseases, accidents, disabilities.

2. Motivate and facilitate needed personal action by the individual patient (as well as by other family members, where appropriate) in cooperation with physicians, other health care professionals, and medical care institutions, in the management of the patient's particular condition.
3. Encourage more efficient, effective, and economic use of the medical care delivery system by providing information and criteria with which individuals can develop a keen awareness and understanding of the system and its processes.
4. Promote citizen participation in the planning and management of health care delivery systems, both community and institutional, by providing information and interpretation, opening up communication channels, and facilitating involvement.

NOTES

1. Miller, L., and Goldstein, J. "More Effective Care of Diabetes Patients in a County Hospital Setting." *New England Journal of Medicine*, June 29, 1972, pp. 1388–91.
2. Levine, P.H., and Britten, A.F. "Supervised Patient Management of Hemophilia." *Annals of Internal Medicine*, No. 78, 1973, pp. 195–202.

3. Avery, C. H., Green, L. W., and Kreider, S. "Reducing Emergency Visits of Asthmatics." Testimony, President's Committee on Health Education. Pittsburgh, Pa., January 11, 1972.
4. Rosenberg, S. G. "Patient Education Leads to Better Care for Heart Patients." HSMHA *Health Reports*, September 1971, pp. 793–802.
5. Egbert, I. D., et al. "Reduction of Postoperative Pain by Encouragement in Instruction of Patients." *New England Journal of Medicine*, April 16, 1964, pp. 825–827.

Appendix E

AHA's Policy and Statement on the Hospital's Responsibility for Health Promotion, House of Delegates, August 28, 1979

Source: Reprinted with the permission of the American Hospital Association, © 1979.

appendix E

POLICY

Hospitals have a responsibility to take a leadership role in helping ensure the good health of their communities. In addition to their primary mission of providing health care and related education to the sick and injured, hospitals have a responsibility to work with others in the community to assess the health status of the community, identify target health areas and population groups for hospital-based and cooperative health promotion programs, develop programs to help upgrade the health in those target areas, ensure that persons who are apparently healthy have access to information about how to stay well and prevent disease, provide appropriate health education programs to aid those persons who choose to alter their personal health behavior or develop a more healthful life style, and establish the hospital within the community as an institution which is concerned about good health as well as one concerned with treating illness.

STATEMENT

Increasing numbers of people are seeking information about their health and making more and more decisions without the direct consultation of physicians or other health professionals.

The American Hospital Association has supported and encouraged this trend toward greater personal responsibility for health in its *Statement on the Provision of Health Services Under National Health Insurance*: "Each individual, to the extent he or she is able, has the personal responsibility for protecting his or her own health . . . " The statement also identifies an active role for health care providers in helping the consumer achieve this goal: "The system should be oriented to the maintenance of personal good health and to the prevention of illness, as well as to the treatment of acute illness" and hospitals should "develop and participate in community-wide health education and information activities to actively encourage responsible decisions about health, as well as responsible use of health services by its comunity." Indeed, hospitals traditionally have been involved in health promotion activities.

HOSPITALS' IMAGE: THE CENTER FOR HEALTH

In many communities, the hospital is identified by the public as the center for health, and thus is looked to as the logical source for all types of information relating to health as well as sickness. It is to hospitals' advantage to encourage this positive image through management support and board level policy. Further, people look to health professionals as exemplars or models to be copied. Thus, hospitals should take a leadership role in providing appropriate health information and education to their communities, and to the employees of the institution.

HOSPITALS AS A CATALYST

Hospitals, physicians, and other health professionals should serve as catalysts to stimulate the interest of, encourage the participation of, and develop strong working relationships with voluntary health agencies, other health provider groups, educational institutions, local businesses and industries, and other groups within the community that influence and/or control resources needed in order to carry out these responsibilities. The fulfillment of these responsibilities will help ensure that patients, hospital employees and community members have the information needed to enable them to make informed choices about their personal health behavior, their life styles, and the environment in which they live, since the responsibility for these decisions rests with the individual.

HEALTH PROMOTION: INFORMED CHOICE

Health promotion (including health information and health education) is the process of fostering awareness, influencing attitudes, and identifying alternatives so that individuals can make informed choices and change their behavior in order to achieve an optimum level of physical and mental health and improve their physical and social environment. Health promotion programs offered by hospitals should facilitate this informed choice, but should not have as their goal forcing specific habits or life style choices (unless it can be demonstrated that an individual's health practices adversely and seriously affect the health of others).

PROTECTING INDIVIDUAL'S RIGHTS

In those areas where it can be demonstrated that the actions of one individual adversely and seriously affect the health of others, such as through alcohol or drug abuse, or sidestream smoke, hospitals have a responsibility to take appropriate steps to protect the rights of the affected individuals within the institutions. For example, hospitals have a responsibility to protect the rights of nonsmoking patients, employees, and visitors within their institution. To the extent feasible, they also have a responsibility to work with others in the community—such as physicians, voluntary health agencies, health provider groups, educational institutions, local businesses and industries, and other interested groups—to make available information on the hazards to others of reckless driving, alcohol and drug abuse, smoking and other harmful practices, and to make available appropriate behavior change programs. As with all hospital services, steps should be taken to assure confidentiality.

LIFE STYLE

Hospitals have long supported the concept of disease-oriented patient education. The phrases "responsible decisions about health" and "maintenance of personal good health," as contained in the *Statement on the Provision of Health Services Under National Health Insurance*, however, imply a role that goes beyond disease related information and take hospitals into the area of life style and personal behavior. (Life style includes such personal choice factors as the use or abuse of alcohol, drugs, tobacco and the automobile, as well as exercise, nutrition and sleep habits.)

COOPERATIVE EFFORTS

In order to ensure the most effective use of community resources, including funding, and to provide the broadest possible benefits from health promotion programs, it is appropriate and necessary for hospitals to work with others in the community to provide information and education about: the value of and techniques for achieving a healthful life style; the potential dangers to the individual and to others from certain personal health habits;

methods to prevent disease; and opportunities for early disease detection and treatment. This may include stimulating, encouraging and working closely with physicians and other health professionals, hospital auxiliaries and volunteers, voluntary health agencies, health provider groups, third-party payers, public health departments, and other interested groups, as well as developing new and stronger health promotion channels through cooperation with school systems, religious organizations, local government, local businesses and industries, and the news media.

COSTS AND HEALTH PROMOTION

Many personal health and life style factors are related to expensive and preventable illnesses and accidents. The Council on Wage and Price Stability stated: "Health education can reduce health care costs in several ways. Education as to proper nutrition and exercise can help reduce the incidence of illness. So too, can counseling services on alcoholism and emotional problem areas reduce the incidence of physiological and mental illness."[1] Thus, health information and education programs relating to life style and personal health behavior are appropriate for institutions concerned about rising costs.

However, financing health promotion activities often poses problems for hospitals, especially in an environment of conscientious cost containment. Experience shows that hospitals are utilizing a wide range of appropriate financing mechanisms to balance their commitments to containing costs. These financing mechanisms include third-party reimbursement, fee-for-service, donations from attendees, contributions and gifts, grants and contracts, and the extensive use of volunteer help.

NOTE

1. *The Complex Puzzle of Rising Health Care Costs: Can The Private Sector Fit It Together?*, a report for the Council on Wage and Price Stability, 1976.

Appendix F

AHA's Policy and Statement on the Hospital's Responsibility for Patient Education Services, House of Delegates, September 1, 1981*

Source: Reprinted with the permission of the American Hospital Association, © 1981.

*Replaces the 1974 Policy Statement: *Role and Responsibilities of Hospitals and Other Health Care Institutions in Personal and Community Education.*

appendix F

POLICY

The Hospital has a responsibility to provide patient education services as an integral part of high-quality, cost-effective care. Patient education services should enable patients, and their families and friends, when appropriate, to make informed decisions about their health; to manage their illnesses; and to implement follow-up care at home. Effective and efficient patient education services require planning and coordination, and responsibility for such planning and coordination should be assigned. The hospital also should provide the necessary staff and financial resources.

STATEMENT

Terms

Health education is the use of the education process to assist individuals to voluntarily adopt or alter behaviors that will improve or maintain their health.

Patient education is used when the health education is directed to persons, and their families and friends, when appropriate, who are either awaiting or undergoing medical treatment.

Planned patient education uses a process that includes conducting a needs assessment, setting objectives, and developing an action plan and the implementation, documentation, and evaluation of that action plan.

Patient education services include a variety of services developed to respond to the education needs of patients and families. These services should include planned activities designed to inform patients about how to use various health care services, to prepare patients for medical procedures, to assist patients to manage their diseases or to use a medical device after discharge, and to modify their behavior in order to promote better health and prevent diseases. These services can incorporate one or a combination of one-to-one instruction, group sessions, a series of classes, and support groups.

Rationale

Hospitals have always provided health information to patients and their families. However, with pressures on hospitals to contain costs while responding to the increased need for patient education services, it is important that hospitals plan and coordinate their patient education services. Planning and coordination allows hospitals to make decisions about patient education services that are appropriate for their patients and resources.

Experience and research have identified several benefits of planned patient education services both to the hospital and to patients.

For the patient, planned patient education services can reduce anxiety, increase ability to make health decisions, and reduce readmissions for chronic diseases.

For the hospital, planned and coordinated patient education can enhance efficient use of hospital services, promote efficient use of education resources, increase physician support through the collaborative development of accurate teaching program content, increase staff satisfaction, increase patient satisfaction with patient services, and increase community support for the hospital.

In addition, the provision of planned and coordinated patient education services assists the hospital to respond to pressures of: accreditation standards for patient education; requirements for informed consent; need for cost efficient use of resources; increased numbers of persons needing education to help manage chronic conditions or information about new diagnostic and treatment services; and increased consumer interest in making health decisions.

Coordination

To meet the various education needs of patients, relatives, or friends in the preadmitting, admitting, inpatient, outpatient, and discharge stages of care, patient education goals and activities should be planned and coordinated at three levels: the entire hospital; specific patient populations, such as those with hypertension or on low sodium diets; and individual patients and families. The education planning process is applied to all three levels.

In order to implement planned, coordinated patient education services, the responsibility should be assigned to a hospital committee, department, or staff person. The responsible individual or group should possess education and management skills and should enable the hospital to implement staff policies and procedures on the roles and responsibilities of persons providing patient education, staff training programs, staff performance evaluations that include patient education activities, documentation of patient education services as part of patient care, and evaluations of patient education services and subsequent implementation of changes in program content.

The coordinating committee, department, or staff person should involve the medical staff and individuals in various hospital departments and hospital committees, as well as selected patients, in making decisions about the content of and methods for conducting patient education services. These decisions help to determine the staff skills, the time, and the space needed to implement patient education services.

Human Resources

The assignment of responsibility for planning and coordination should enable the hospital and its staff to use their time and skills more effectively and efficiently. Although the responsibility for planning and coordinating patient education services is assigned, direct care staff, including physicians, nurses, dieticians, pharmacists, and others, are involved in patient education as part of the delivery of high-quality patient care services. Other individuals in the hospital such as librarians, patient representatives, and selected patients and family members can assist in the development and provision of patient education services. Trained volunteers and auxiliaries also can be a valuable resource.

Financial Resources

In order to implement planned coordinated patient education services, hospitals should provide the necessary staff and financial resources. Expenses for providing patient education services directly related to patient care should be treated as financial requirements under third-party agreements.

Community Resources

Community agencies may be a source of funding and they also may have patient education materials, staff expertise, and patient education services. To assist patients needing patient education after discharge, as well as to expand their patient education resources and those of their community, hospitals should work with these agencies to refer patients, to develop cooperative activities, and to share resources.

Hospitals also should explore the feasibility of sharing and utilizing patient education resources with hospitals, hospital associations, and other health care settings.

Appendix G

A Self-Study Guide for Hospital Health Education

appendix G

	YES	NO	COMMENTS
INSTITUTIONAL			
Has a community needs assessment been done?			
Has an institutional needs assessment been done?			
Are there policy statements or board level commitments to the program?			
Are goals, objectives, and plans clearly written and disseminated?			
Are measures taken to promote the program to hospital staff?			
Is appropriate publicity made available to the community?			
Is there a coordinator with responsibility for the program?			
Does the coordinator have adequate training in health education?			
Is staffing adequate? Are measures being taken to correct staff deficiencies?			
Are the job descriptions for health education staff accurate and current?			

	YES	NO	COMMENTS
Is there an institutional planning committee?			
Is there a community advisory commmittee?			
Have cooperative relationships been established with other area hospitals?			
Is there appropriate inhouse administrative support?			
Is there adequate medical support?			
Are programs available to the patient and family?			
Are programs available to outpatients?			
Are programs available to community members?			
Are programs available for hospital staff?			
Is there adequate space for classes, group discussions, etc.?			
Is there adequate media equipment and facilities?			
Is there an adequate budget for teaching aids, books, journals?			
Is there adequate storage space for educational materials?			
Is there a budget item specific for staff development?			
Have external funds been sought to supplement the budget?			
Are educational records a permanent part of the medical records?			

	YES	*NO*	*COMMENTS*
Is the record keeping system adequate to measure effort, efficiency, effect, and impact?			
Is there any research being done in the program on specific approaches, target groups, etc.?			
Are articles published or presentations made to professional groups sharing your experience?			
Have both strengths and weaknesses of the program been identified and short-range strategies been designed to accommodate them?			
PROGRAMMATIC Does the title identify the general content of the program?			
Is the specific target group for whom this program is intended identified?			
Do the objectives describe expected learning objectives or outcomes which can be measured and evaluated?			
Are objectives written in terms of what the client will do rather than what the staff will do?			
Are there specific objectives in the cognitive, affective, and psychomotor domains?			
Is the amount of scheduled teaching time specified for content units?			
Is the content specified in sufficient detail for other staff members to utilize if necessary?			

	YES	NO	COMMENTS
Are the teaching methods and content appropriate for the learner population?			
Are teaching methods detailed sufficiently so as to be useable by other staff?			
Are teaching methods appropriate to the learning domains?			
Is the time and place of teaching identified?			
Are appropriate teaching aids specified and readily available?			
Are hand-outs evaluated periodically?			
Are procedures clear for who is responsible for evaluating patient readiness?			
Is there a written tool to assist staff in assessing the learning needs of clients?			
Is responsibility fixed as to who will assess patient learnings and record it?			
Do the guidelines specify who will be responsible for recording data on patient learnings?			
Are available community agencies identified for referral?			
Does discharge planning occur for all patients needing it?			

Appendix H

A Selected Bibliography

appendix H

American Hospital Association. *Implementing Patient Education in the Hospital*. Chicago: American Hospital Association, 1979.

American Hospital Association. *Hospital In Patient Education: Survey Finding and Analysis*. Chicago: American Hospital Association, 1980.

Czerwinski, Barbara S. *Manual of Patient Education for Cardiopulmonary Dysfunction*. St. Louis: C. V. Mosby Company, 1980.

Green, Lawrence; Kreuter, Marshall W.; Deeds, Sigrid G.; and Partridge, Kay B. *Health Education Planning, A Diagnostic Approach*. Palo Alto, Ca.: Mayfield Publishing Company, 1980.

Lazes, Peter M., ed. *The Handbook of Health Education*. Rockville, Md.: Aspen Systems Corporation, 1979.

Narrow, Barbara W. *Patient Teaching in Nursing Practice: A Patient and Family-Centered Approach*. New York: John Wiley and Sons, 1979.

McCormick, Rose-Marie Duda and Gilson-Parkevich, Tamar. *Patient and Family Education: Tools, Techniques, and Theory*. New York: John Wiley and Sons, 1979.

Pritchett, Sue. *Patient, Family and Community Health Education: Design and Management of Hospital Based Programs*. Atlanta: Pritchett and Hull Associates, 1977.

Redman, Barbara Klug. *The Process of Patient Teaching in Nursing*. 4th rev. ed. St. Louis: C. V. Mosby Company, 1980.

Ross, Helen S. and Mico, Paul R. *Theory and Practice in Health Education*. Palo Alto, Ca.: Mayfield Publishing Co., 1980.

Squyres, Wendy D., ed. *Patient Education: An Inquiry into the State of the Art*. New York: Springer Publishing Co., 1980.

Zander, Karen S.; Bower, Kathleen A.; Foster, Susan D.; Towson, Marilynn C.; Wermuth, Mara Ruments; and Waldum, Karyl M. *Practical Manual For Patient Teaching*, St. Louis: C. V. Mosby, 1978.

Journals and Newsletters

Focal Points, Bureau of Health Education, Public Health Service, Center for Disease Control, Atlanta, GA 30333.

Health Education Quarterly, Society for Public Health Education, 703 Market Street, San Francisco, CA 94103.

Health Values: Achieving High Level Wellness, Charles Slack Inc., 6900 Grove Road, Thorofare, NJ 08086.

Hospitals, American Hospital Association, 840 North Lakeshore Drive, Chicago, IL 60611.

Patient Counseling and Health Education, Excerta Medica, PO Box 3085, Princeton, NJ 08540.

Promoting HEALTH, American Hospital Association, 840 North Lakeshore Drive, Chicago, IL 60611

Index

About the Author

DONALD BRECKON was born, raised, and educated in Michigan. He has a Bachelor's Degree in Education and a Master of Arts Degree in Health Education from Central Michigan University. He has a Masters of Public Health with emphasis in Health Education from the University of Michigan and a Ph.D. from Michigan State University in Adult and Continuing Education. He was a 1979–80 Postdoctoral Fellow in Academic Administration with the American Council on Education.

Dr. Breckon has been on the faculty at Central Michigan University since 1963, as an Instructor, Assistant Professor, and Associate Professor, and currently holds the rank of Professor of Health Education. He also serves as Assistant Dean of Health, Physical Education, Recreation, and Athletics.

He developed the undergraduate and graduate programs in Public Health Education and in Patient Education, which he currently directs. He has published extensively in the journals of the discipline and is actively involved in consultation and inservice training in hospital health education.

Dr. Breckon is married and has four teenage daughters. He is active in university and community activities.